Praise for Professor

BUMP IT UP

'I am absolutely delighted that here, at last, is the definitive guide to *what*, *how much*, and *when* you should exercise, as well as how to mentally prepare yourself for this very important time in your life. And no one is better than Greg at that! He is such a fantastic motivator.'
Davina McCall, author, presenter, fitness expert and mum

'Exercise has always been an important part of my life including through my pregnancies. Exercise had an incredibly positive effect during my pregnancies and helped in my return to full fitness and becoming European Champion following the birth of my daughter. Unfortunately, there is a real lack of good advice on exercise and pregnancy; Greg's new book provides a comprehensive exercise guide pre-, during, and post-pregnancy that is invaluable for all mums and mums-to-be.'
Jo Pavey MBE, European Gold medallist and mum

'For me exercising while being pregnant was so important. It was about feeling energized, helped me carry the extra weight and helped my body bounce a bit quicker back into shape afterwards. Exercising definitely helped and supported me through my pregnancy! It's great that Greg has written a book to support mums-to-be in staying active through pregnancy.'
Rebecca Adlington OBE, double Olympic gold and bronze medallist and mum

'I loved being active while pregnant. For me it was really important because I had quite bad day sickness and it really helped make me feel settled and balanced. Also I'm convinced being fitter made the first few weeks easier. Greg's book provides fantastic support to guide your exercise throughout pregnancy.'
Baroness Tanni Grey-Thompson DBE, DL, Paralympic gold, silver and bronze medallist, world record holder and mum

www.penguin.co.uk

'I strongly believe that gentle safe exercise during pregnancy makes you not only feel better physically, it helps you mentally too. Happy, fit "mummy to be" equals happy birth for baby.'
Denise Van Outen, actress, presenter and mum

'I was exercising a lot before pregnancy and so it was important that I didn't just suddenly stop when I became pregnant – which wouldn't have been good for my body. I continued to run until six months, at which point I listened to my body and knew it was time to stop. Women mustn't be scared to exercise when pregnant as it's so beneficial to their emotional and physical wellbeing and will really benefit them in the early months with their new-born. Greg's new book provides a wonderful companion for mums-to-be.'
Sally Gunnell OBE, Olympic gold medallist, world record holder and mum

BUMP IT UP

The dynamic, flexible exercise and
healthy eating plan for before,
during and after pregnancy

Professor Greg Whyte OBE

BANTAM PRESS

LONDON · NEW YORK · TORONTO · SYDNEY · AUCKLAND

The information and advice in this book are intended as a general guide in relation to the specific subjects addressed. They are not intended as a substitute for medical advice. Do not begin any exercise programme or undertake any self-treatment without first seeking professional guidance from your GP or a qualified healthcare practitioner. So far as the author is aware, the information given is correct and up-to-date as at the time of publication. The author and publishers disclaim, as far as the law allows, any liability arising directly or indirectly from the use, or misuse, of the information contained in this book.

TRANSWORLD PUBLISHERS
61–63 Uxbridge Road, London W5 5SA
www.penguin.co.uk

Transworld is part of the Penguin Random House group of companies
whose addresses can be found at global.penguinrandomhouse.com

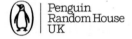

Penguin
Random House
UK

First published in Great Britain in 2016 by Bantam Press
an imprint of Transworld Publishers

A CIP catalogue record for this book
is available from the British Library.

ISBN 9780593077481

Typeset in 10.5/15 pt Nofret Light by Jouve (UK), Milton Keynes
Printed and bound in Great Britain by Clays Ltd, Bungay, Suffolk

Penguin Random House is committed to a sustainable
future for our business, our readers and our planet. This book
is made from Forest Stewardship Council® certified paper.

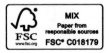

MIX
Paper from
responsible sources
FSC® C018179

1 3 5 7 9 10 8 6 4 2

About the Author

Professor Greg Whyte OBE is a world-leading performance scientist and physical-activity expert, who has spent over two decades enhancing the quality of life of a broad range of people – from Olympic champions, to cancer patients, celebrities and first-time mums. A father of three, he has helped not only his own wife but a huge number of mums, including celebrity mums, optimize their pregnancy, and the delivery and early years of their children.

Greg is a Professor of Sport and Exercise Science at Liverpool John Moores University and Director of the Centre of Health and Human Performance on London's Harley Street, where he runs a specialist exercise, nutrition and lifestyle clinic for pregnancy. He is also a regular media contributor on the topic of exercise and pregnancy, as well as other specialist areas of exercise and performance. Greg is also the author of *Achieve the Impossible*. For more information on Greg Whyte and his work, see his website at www.gregwhyte.com.

To Penny, my wife, my love and the best mummy our three
beautiful children, Maya, Elise and Mitchell, could ever wish for

Contents

Foreword

When I was clubbing and dancing four nights a week for six hours each night, I didn't need to train or follow an exercise plan. I was fit, active and had bags of energy. But after I had my first baby, Holly, I hadn't got rid of my baby weight before I got preggers with my second baby! Anyhoo . . .

With my second pregnancy, I just ballooned. I was absolutely enormous, and there was a severe danger that even my Crocs wouldn't fit me! But I decided to do something positive about this and started exercising while I was pregnant with Tilly. I am so glad I did, and I can honestly say I never looked back. I took a very sensible approach, telling myself, 'Nice and easy does it . . . but DO it!!!'

Greg and I have often talked about the sketchy and sometimes contradictory advice that is out there for pregnant women, which can be very confusing. So I am absolutely delighted that here, at last, is the definitive guide to what, how much, and when you should exercise, as well as how to prepare yourself mentally for this important time in your life. And no one is better than Greg at that! He is such a fantastic motivator.

With *Bump It Up*, in addition to guiding you through the exercise plans for each trimester, Greg and his team provide invaluable advice on nutrition and offer some truly yummy recipes, menu ideas and information on how critical a healthy lifestyle can be if you want to enhance your pregnancy journey from conception through to life as a new mummy.

I would literally walk over hot coals for this man because he got me through the toughest experience of my life, my Sport Relief challenge. I know that when you have your great pregnancy and delivery, you'll want to walk over hot coals for him too!

Davina McCall

Introduction

I am delighted to welcome you to *Bump It Up*, a safe and effective exercise, nutrition and lifestyle programme. While we traditionally think of pregnancy as the nine-month period from conception to birth, it is clear that it is in fact a much longer journey, starting from the path to successful conception and carrying on through the three trimesters of pregnancy and, finally, to the post-partum period and beyond.

Designed to accompany you on your entire pregnancy journey, *Bump It Up* begins with your personal Fertility Lifestyle Programme, a plan devised to optimize your chances of conception. Once you've successfully conceived, the next chapters in the book focus on the importance of exercise and nutrition during pregnancy and provide fully illustrated, easy-to-follow exercise plans for each of the three trimesters. Finally, I've provided detailed guidance on exercise and lifestyle during the post-partum period and beyond – all you need to know about how to look after yourself during this important phase of your life. In short, this chapter is all about *you*!

To complement the exercise programmes, included here is an overview on the important role nutrition plays in our lives – particularly during pregnancy – together with advice on how to achieve a healthy, balanced lifestyle, and essential guidance on what to eat and what to avoid from pre-conception right the way through to the post-partum period. As an added bonus, there is a range of delicious, healthy recipes that have been designed to include an array of nutrients that are particularly beneficial during pregnancy. I hope you will enjoy these simple, stress-free recipes and make them part of your pregnancy journey.

I wish you luck and hope you find *Bump It Up* to be the perfect exercise, nutrition and lifestyle companion for a happy and healthy pregnancy.

1

Your Personal Fertility Lifestyle Programme

Infertility affects a large number of couples (up to 15 per cent of those trying to conceive) and can be an extremely traumatic and stressful experience. Irrespective of age, weight, fitness or any other lifestyle factor, there are sadly some couples who are unable to conceive. The only approach we can take is to do our best to increase the chances of conception. The following chapter details those elements of our lifestyles that can be controlled by our behaviour and examines how best to make positive changes to optimize fertility.

Lifestyles and fertility

It is only recently that we have begun to understand the pivotal role that lifestyle factors play in fertility, particularly in the development of infertility. Lifestyle factors are those habits and behaviours that we control through our own actions and we all understand the impact of many of these on our overall health and well-being – such as the negative effects of smoking, inactivity and excessive alcohol consumption. But now we are also beginning to understand how these poor lifestyle choices may impact upon fertility.

Recent evidence has shown that a large number of lifestyle factors, such as smoking, poor nutrition, alcohol, caffeine, high body weight (fat mass), lack of exercise, psychological stress, illicit drugs and environmental and occupational toxins, can have substantial effects on fertility. What is very important to remember is that these are all modifiable aspects, which you have the power to control. You can take active steps to enhance your and your partner's fertility and improve your chances of conception.

Of course, improving one's fertility is not an exact science and only a small number of scientific studies have examined the role of lifestyle factors in improving the chances of becoming pregnant. What is clear, however, is that closely examining your own habits and designing a 'fertility lifestyle programme' tailored to your own personal needs is important in optimizing your fertility.

There is no 'one-size-fits-all' solution when it comes to lifestyle factors and there is often a graded scale of the benefits to be accrued from making changes. For example, simply reducing your intake of alcohol and caffeine, rather than cutting them out completely, can improve your fertility, while for smoking the advice is clear – stop it completely. In addition, changes can be made in different directions. For example, you should increase the amount of exercise you do and reduce your stress levels – and exercise can often contribute to stress reduction.

There are, of course, limits to the benefits that can be gained from lifestyle changes and it is rarely a simple matter of 'if a little is good, then more is better'. Take exercise for example: research suggests that regular workouts improve reproductive function in women who exercise at a moderate intensity for 30 minutes or more daily, reducing the risk of infertility associated with ovulation disorders. In contrast, excessive amounts of high-intensity exercise may actually lower fertility, particularly if the menstrual cycle is negatively affected. So getting the balance right and designing your own 'fertility lifestyle programme' is crucial to improving your chances of getting pregnant.

Factors affecting female fertility

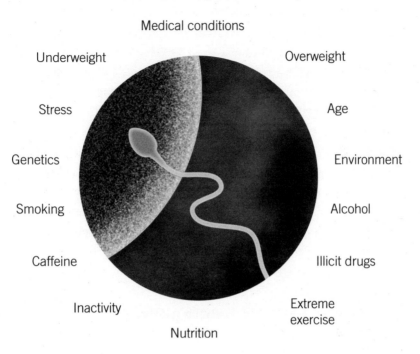

Medical conditions

Underweight

Overweight

Stress

Age

Genetics

Environment

Smoking

Alcohol

Caffeine

Illicit drugs

Inactivity

Extreme
exercise

Nutrition

It's a weighty matter!

We know that body weight plays an important role in fertility and, in particular, avoiding excess weight appears to be central to optimizing your chances of conception. Maintaining a healthy weight is where diet and exercise come in. The target weight for most women appears to be a normal BMI (18.5–24.9). However, it is not all about your BMI, which only takes into account height and weight. Body composition, which is the combination of muscle mass and fat mass, is particularly important. Research suggests that ovulation is impaired if fat mass drops below 15 per cent or if it exceeds 35 per cent of total body mass. Exercise plays a key role in increasing muscle mass and reducing fat mass, so a good combination of diet and exercise can put you in the right fertility zone.

Of course, it's not just about being overweight. Men who are underweight (with a BMI of less than 18.5) have lower sperm counts than those who have a normal BMI. For women, being underweight and having very low body fat is linked to disruption of the menstrual cycle and ovarian dysfunction. This situation is made worse when your BMI falls below 17. Eating disorders such as anorexia nervosa and bulimia are linked to irregular menses (oligomenorrhoea) or loss of menses (amenorrhoea) and infertility, and during pregnancy are associated with negative impacts on maternal and foetal well-being. If you have, or suspect you have, an eating disorder, it is important that you seek advice and support from your healthcare team.

How much exercise is enough?

There is a sweet spot for fertility when it comes to exercise – and it is definitely not a 'more is better' approach! Excessive exercise can create a negative energy balance, particularly when calorie consumption is restricted, and this can have a harmful impact on your reproductive system. It is not uncommon for elite female athletes, particularly endurance athletes, to experience irregular periods or loss of menstruation. The message here is that a little is good but a lot may be problematic. As with most things in life, a balanced, sensible approach to exercise is the way forward. Indeed, evidence suggests that 4 hours of moderate-intensity exercise each week may be the tipping point beyond which increased exercise duration and/or intensity may negatively impact on fertility. If you exercise excessively (and you really should not), you should ensure that you are optimizing your nutrition (calorie intake) to reduce any potentially detrimental effects.

Men who are moderately active (around 3 hours per week) at a moderate intensity have a higher sperm count, sperm speed and better sperm morphology (shape) than either highly active men or elite athletes. What type of exercise men do may also be important; research shows that those who cycle for long periods each week have a lower sperm count.

Importantly, as mentioned, it appears that the interaction between exercise and nutrition is the key to optimizing fertility. Using a combination of exercise and calorie restriction to create a negative energy balance, where your energy expenditure is greater than your energy consumption (food), and to reduce weight and fat mass appears to have positive outcomes for obese women (and men) when it comes to fertility. At the other end of the scale, for women who are underweight or who suffer from an eating disorder, it is important to address the low-calorie state of their diet and add moderate levels of exercise to optimize fertility. For normal-weight women and men, ensuring an energy balance with moderate amounts of exercise combined with a calorie-matched healthy, balanced diet has the most positive effect on fertility.

You are what you eat!

We all know that diet plays a central role in our general health and well-being. But what you may not know is that modifying the macronutrients (carbohydrates, proteins and fats) and micronutrients (vitamins and minerals) in your diet could have a positive effect on your fertility.

For women, the consumption of trans-fats and excessive animal protein has been shown to reduce fertility. In contrast, complex carbohydrates, such as vegetable-based proteins and vegetables rich in iron (such as spinach, broccoli, kale and mushrooms), are linked to improved fertility. Reactive Oxygen Species (ROS) are by-products of energy production in all cells in the body, which, in excess, can lead to oxidative stress, resulting in cell damage and dysfunction. Your body's natural defences include antioxidants that scavenge (consume) ROS. In addition to these natural defences, you can increase your antioxidant level through your diet (by including foods such as blueberries, avocados, kidney beans and dark leafy greens), or by taking supplements such as multivitamins. Evidence suggests that women who consume foods rich in antioxidants and who supplement with multivitamins have improved fertility.

And it's not all about you! Your partner can positively impact his fertility by making a variety of changes. In men, an overabundance of ROS can reduce sperm motility (movement) and alter its DNA. Research demonstrates that men consuming antioxidants, including vitamins B, C and E, have improved sperm motility, conception and birth rates. In addition, consuming a diet rich in complex carbohydrates, and fruit and vegetables high in fibre, folate (green leafy vegetables) and lycopene (tomatoes) has been shown to improve semen quality. As with women, a diet high in trans-fats and protein appears to be detrimental to fertility.

Caffeine kicks!

The link between caffeine and fertility is not fully understood. A small number of studies have suggested that high caffeine consumption (more than 500mg per day – about 4 or 5 cups; although upper limits as low as 100mg are considered by some to be problematic) may affect ovulation and the time it takes to conceive. In addition, there is evidence that caffeine can negatively impact the foetus during pregnancy. Although further studies are needed in this area, given the evidence so far you should consider cutting down on your caffeine intake, particularly of coffee, tea and fizzy drinks. If you are at all concerned, stop your caffeine intake altogether.

Just a little tipple!

There is definitely a link between alcohol consumption and infertility. However, it is not clear how much is too much. It does appear that there is a 'dose-dependent response'; in other words, the more you drink, the more likely you are to have fertility problems. The reason for this altered fertility appears to be the detrimental effect alcohol has on your hormones, in particular lowering levels of oestrogen and follicle stimulating hormone (FSH), which leads to the suppression of ovulation. In men, alcohol consumption is linked to shrinking of the testicles and a decreased sperm count and motility. While many believe that alcohol is a magic love potion, it does in fact reduce libido! In general, the best advice is to reduce your alcohol consumption to a moderate level (no more than 14 units for men and 7 units for women in a week, and no more than 4 units for men, 3 units for women in a single session). Better still, aim for even lower than this or stop altogether to improve your chances of conception. Remember, less is definitely more when it comes to alcohol!

Fertility up in smoke!

It's not rocket science! Smoking is bad for your health and bad for your fertility. There is no safe limit where smoking is concerned; every drag you take floods your lungs with over 4,000 dangerous chemicals and has a negative impact on your health and fertility. Don't kid yourself that it won't affect you because you are only an 'occasional smoker'; research has shown that even light smokers have reduced fertility.

Smoking reduces ovarian function and ovarian reserve (the capacity of the ovary to provide eggs that can be fertilized). Smoking can also cause menstrual dysfunction and changes in hormones such as progesterone and follicle stimulating hormone. And it doesn't just affect you; evidence shows that men who smoke have increased sperm DNA damage, decreased sperm counts and motility, lower semen volume and fertilizing capacity. There really is only one course of action – STOP SMOKING.

Stressed out!

Stress is not always a bad thing, but when you are highly stressed over prolonged periods your stress hormones (adrenaline and cortisol) are chronically elevated, which can negatively affect ovulation. For most of us, stress comes in three forms: physical, psychological and sociological. These three types rarely operate in isolation. For example, stress at work (sociological stress) can result in psychological stress (anxiety disorders, depression, etc.), which in turn leads to physical changes, such as elevated levels of stress hormones.

For men, excessive stress, which is often associated with anxiety and depression, negatively affects gonadal function, and reduces testosterone and other key hormones, such as luteinizing hormone. These changes have been shown to reduce sperm count and sperm motility, and cause problems with sperm production and shape.

The double whammy here is that infertility in itself is stressful. Our hopes and dreams of parenthood, not to mention the pressure from our friends, family and society at large to have children, can be overwhelming when you are struggling to conceive. On top of all this, the strain of medical appointments, tests, associated costs, and failures to conceive can make infertility one of the most stressful experiences in life. Add general life pressures to this toxic mix and you have the perfect storm for long-term infertility. That's why it is so important that you make every effort to reduce your levels of physical, psychological and sociological stress when you are trying to conceive.

There are a whole variety of strategies that you should explore if you feel this is an issue in your life. Examples include meditation, mindfulness and cognitive behavioural therapy. Importantly, exercise is a fabulous stress buster. In addition to the physical benefits, the release of endorphins (the 'happy hormones') during exercise not only improves mood but also reduces anxiety and stress. Exercising with family and friends, including attending classes, provides a wonderful environment for support and fun that can ease life's worries and promote relaxation, which may in turn improve fertility.

Your fertility lifestyle programme

As we have seen, and to recap, there are a number of lifestyle factors that can affect your fertility and, while making the changes suggested in this chapter will not guarantee conception, there is no doubt that you have the power to improve your chances if you make the right lifestyle choices.

When it comes to your size, your target should be a normal BMI (18.5–24.9). As discussed, being overweight disturbs hormone production and ovulation, thus reducing fertility. But so too does being underweight, which is linked to menstrual dysfunction and impaired fertility.

Taking regular exercise and eating a healthy diet are the most effective methods for controlling your body weight and they can also enhance your fertility. Regular, moderate-duration (3 to 4 hours per week), moderate-intensity exercise, combined with a healthy, balanced diet targeting specific macro- and micronutrients has been shown to improve fertility for both men and women.

Stopping smoking and cutting down on your alcohol and caffeine intake should be an essential part of your fertility lifestyle programme.

Reducing stress, whatever its cause, should be a priority during this very important time. Think about your fertility lifestyle programme as a team event; make sure you surround yourself with family and friends who fully support your goal. And don't forget to stay in regular contact with your healthcare team to make sure you are on track to optimize your fertility.

	YOUR FERTILITY LIFESTYLE PROGRAMME CHECKLIST	
	You	**Your partner**
Weight	BMI of 18.5 to 24.9 Fat mass of 15 to 35 per cent	BMI of 18.5 to 24.9 Fat mass of 15 to 20 per cent
Exercise	3 to 4 hours of moderate-intensity exercise	3 to 4 hours of moderate-intensity exercise
Diet	Focus on complex carbohydrates, vegetable-based proteins, vegetables rich in iron, and fruit and vegetables high in antioxidants. Consider a daily multivitamin supplement. Avoid trans-fats and excessive amounts of animal protein.	Focus on complex carbohydrates, and fruit and vegetables high in fibre, folate (i.e. green leafy vegetables) and lycopene (i.e. tomatoes). Avoid trans-fats and excessive amounts of animal protein.
Caffeine	Less than 500mg per day (4 to 5 cups) – the lower the better.	Support your partner in reducing caffeine consumption.
Alcohol	No more than 7 units per week, and no more than 3 units in a single session. Less is more!	No more than 14 units per week, and no more than 4 units in a single session. Less is more!
Smoking	STOP Avoid smoky environments.	STOP Avoid smoky environments.

	You	Your partner
Pesticides	Wash fruit and vegetables thoroughly. Consider a move to organic.	Wash fruit and vegetables thoroughly. Consider a move to organic.
Stress	Evaluate your stress levels carefully and make the necessary adjustments to home and work life to reduce pressure. Use the available interventions, including exercise, to manage your stress.	Evaluate your stress levels carefully and make the necessary adjustments to home and work life to reduce pressure. Use the available interventions, including exercise, to manage your stress.
Clothing		Avoid prolonged wearing of tight underwear and trousers that increase testicular temperature. Consider changing to 100 per cent cotton underwear.
Illicit drugs	STOP	STOP
Fertility lifestyle programme team	Surround yourself with friends and family who support your goals.	Surround yourself with friends and family who support your goals.

FAQs

Does age matter when it comes to fertility?

Unfortunately, yes. As we age, the fertility levels in both men and women decrease. Research suggests that for women under the age of 30, the chance of conceiving may be over 70 per cent. However, over 36 years of age, it may drop to closer to 40 per cent. One of the main reasons for this is the declining quantity and quality of a woman's eggs as she ages.

For men, the age-related fall in testosterone leads to a decreasing volume and motility of semen, together with increasing DNA damage to sperm. But all is not lost! By making positive changes to all the lifestyle factors covered in this chapter, you can improve your fertility and increase your chances of conception.

My partner loves wearing tight pants but can they be too tight?

Increasing the temperature of the scrotum can have a negative impact on a man's fertility by reducing the production of sperm (spermatogenesis) and negatively affecting a host of factors from the motility to the shape of sperm. Wearing tight pants and trousers, particularly in hot conditions, increases the temperature of the scrotum. As only around a 4°C increase is required to negatively affect fertility, it's easy to see how prolonged wearing of snug underwear can impact on your chances of conception. The answer is simple: let it all hang out! Avoid wearing tight clothing on a continual basis, wear loose underwear – preferably 100 per cent cotton, which is a 'breathable fabric' – and trousers as much as possible, and go commando at night!

Can smoking marijuana cause infertility?

Marijuana contains cannabinoids, which have been shown to reduce fertility. Cannabinoids attach to receptors in the uterus in women and the vas deferens (part of the reproductive system) in men, which results in altered function.

In women, cannabinoids have been linked to changes in hormone regulation that negatively impact on fertility. In men, cannabinoids have been linked to reduced testosterone production, sperm count and sperm motility. As marijuana is also illegal, the best advice is not to use it in any form and avoid environments where it is used if you want to improve your chances of conception. It goes without saying that the same advice holds true for other illicit drugs, including cocaine.

Can pesticides used in food production affect fertility?

There is some evidence to show that pesticides can impair fertility in a number of ways. In women, it appears that pesticides may affect your hormones and lead to irregular menses. In men, there is some evidence to suggest that pesticides decrease semen quality, alter semen DNA, cause erectile dysfunction and decrease libido. The most obvious place we come into contact with pesticides is in our food, so make sure you wash your food thoroughly before eating, and consider changing to organic produce in order to reduce your exposure to harmful chemicals.

PREGNANCY TRIVIA

You're not alone

Approximately 10 to 15 per cent of couples are affected by infertility.

Meds

As well as illicit drug use, some prescribed medications can have a negative effect on fertility in both men and women. Speak to your GP about possible side effects of medications that you are taking and how you might enhance your fertility. An important note: never stop taking prescribed medication without talking to your GP first.

Hold that call!

A number of recent studies have demonstrated the negative effects on fertility of the electromagnetic radiation emitted by mobile phones! One study suggested that men who carry their phone on their belts or in their pockets are more likely to have decreased sperm motility. While the jury is out on this subject, it might be worth popping your phone in your jacket pocket!

What's up, Doc?

Looking after your health and speaking to your doctor if you are worried about your or your partner's fertility has been shown to improve your chances of conception. For example, keeping to your appointments for cervical screening tests or seeking treatment for sexual dysfunctions and infections have been shown to improve fertility. As always, it is usually men who are reluctant to seek help and support; so, as well as looking after yourself, give him a nudge!

Work it out!

Even working long hours (more than 32 hours per week) has been shown to reduce fertility due to its association with increased stress levels. Finding the right work–life balance could be more important than you think. So take a close look at how hard and how long you work, to ensure you are not putting your fertility goals at risk.

2

Pregnancy and Exercise

We all know that exercise is wholly beneficial for our health and quality of life, a fact that remains true throughout pregnancy and beyond. Although your body will undergo a host of changes during this exciting nine-month period, there are very few instances where exercise is not recommended for otherwise healthy mothers experiencing low-risk pregnancies. The benefits of exercise are broad in scope, ranging from improved physical and mental health to enhanced emotional well-being and even social integration, as outlined in the diagram overleaf.

What is exercise?

This may seem like a blindingly obvious question but essentially exercise is any activity that requires physical effort and which is carried out to sustain, maintain or improve health and fitness. In fact, any activity that causes an increase in your heart rate can be considered to be exercise. So whether you're doing the housework, gardening, playing football, walking, jogging, cycling or swimming – they can all be deemed useful exercise. It is particularly important

Physical, mental, emotional and social benefits of exercise

PHYSICAL	MENTAL
Improved quality of life	*Reduced depression*
Improved fitness	Reduced anxiety
Better posture	Reduced stress
Better balance	**Better sleep**
Reduced incidence of illness	Increased cognitive function
Weight control	*Improved energy levels*
Stronger muscles	*Relaxation*
Stronger bones	

SOCIAL	EMOTIONAL
Meet new people	*Increased happiness*
Build social skills	**Increased positive mood**
Strengthen relationships	**Better self-esteem**
Spend more time with friends and family	*Increased self-confidence*
	Improved feelings of success
	Reduced feelings of sadness
	Lower anger and tension

to view exercise in this way during pregnancy, when less structured forms of activity, such as housework or gardening, can easily lead you to exceed the recommended intensity level (see page 28). Don't disregard anything you do that involves physical activity and which increases your heart rate, as it all counts as part of an active lifestyle during pregnancy.

How much is enough?

The recommended amount of exercise for optimal health and well-being is 150 minutes of moderate-intensity activity per week, plus two strength-based sessions. These recommendations also hold true during pregnancy. However, given the increased stress placed upon specific parts of your body during pregnancy and delivery, there are some additional elements you need to add to your exercise programme to ensure you optimize your health and well-being during this special nine-month period. In particular, the additional stress pregnancy places on your core and pelvic floor muscles requires very specific attention to core strength and stability, and pelvic floor exercises pre-, during and post-partum.

While this appears to be a very simple message, there is often a great deal of confusion regarding the type, intensity, duration and frequency of exercise during pregnancy and post-partum. Some elements of your exercise routine will remain constant throughout your pregnancy, while others will change according to the particular stage you are at. You will also have an increased level of concern about what is safe and what isn't during this life-changing period. In this chapter, we will tackle some of the generic issues surrounding exercise and pregnancy, leaving the trimester-specific issues for the following chapters.

Why is pregnancy a special case when it comes to exercise?

As soon as you become pregnant, a whole host of changes begin to take place within your body and this process of transformation will continue over the entire course of the next nine months and beyond. These changes occur primarily to secure the well-being of your baby as he or she develops, right through to the moment of delivery. But some persist for prolonged periods of time post-partum. For example, cardiovascular (heart and blood vessels) changes start to occur within five weeks of conception and are maintained until approximately a year after birth! What is important to remember here is that many of the changes will affect what, when and how you exercise throughout your pregnancy and well into the post-partum period.

Many of the important physical and emotional changes that take place during pregnancy are controlled by key hormones. Levels of hormones including progesterone, oestrogen, human chorionic gonadotrophin (HCG) and human placental lactogen all increase during pregnancy. Another important hormone is relaxin, levels of which peak at 12 weeks and then again prior to delivery. This hormone is responsible for a softening of the connective tissue and ligaments, leading to an increased laxity of your joints (a subject we will return to on a regular basis throughout this book).

There are a number of changes to your cardiovascular system during pregnancy. The amount of blood your heart pumps each minute (termed 'cardiac output') increases by around 40 per cent. This is achieved by an increased resting heart rate during pregnancy and an increase in the amount of blood your heart pumps with each beat (termed 'stroke volume'), which occur at the same time as an overall increase in blood volume, which can expand by up to 50 per cent. To avoid a dramatic rise in blood pressure, the increased level of progesterone you produce during pregnancy leads to a reduction in the resistance of your blood vessels. Importantly, as a result of these changes, there is a significant rise in blood flow to your uterus. In the blood, elevations in lipids, cholesterol, calcium, phosphorous and potassium are commonly observed.

Progesterone is also responsible for dramatic changes to your respiratory system that occur very early in pregnancy, even before the growth of your bump is sufficient to impact on your breathing. In response to your changing hormones, your lower ribs move outwards by up to 5cm and your main respiratory muscle, your diaphragm, located at the bottom of your ribcage, moves upwards by around 4cm. Combined, these changes lead to an increase in the

Changes in your body during pregnancy

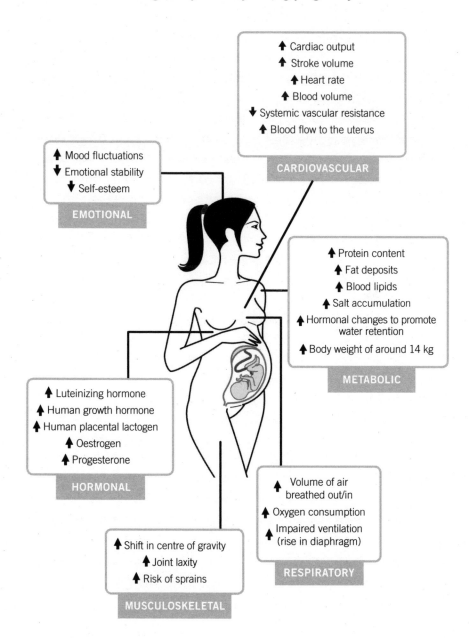

↑ Cardiac output
↑ Stroke volume
↑ Heart rate
↑ Blood volume
↓ Systemic vascular resistance
↑ Blood flow to the uterus

CARDIOVASCULAR

↑ Mood fluctuations
↓ Emotional stability
↓ Self-esteem

EMOTIONAL

↑ Protein content
↑ Fat deposits
↑ Blood lipids
↑ Salt accumulation
↑ Hormonal changes to promote water retention
↑ Body weight of around 14 kg

METABOLIC

↑ Luteinizing hormone
↑ Human growth hormone
↑ Human placental lactogen
↑ Oestrogen
↑ Progesterone

HORMONAL

↑ Volume of air breathed out/in
↑ Oxygen consumption
↑ Impaired ventilation (rise in diaphragm)

RESPIRATORY

↑ Shift in centre of gravity
↑ Joint laxity
↑ Risk of sprains

MUSCULOSKELETAL

work of breathing, which is often amplified as your pregnancy progresses and your uterus increases in size, pushing up on your diaphragm.

During pregnancy, metabolic (energy production) processes change. In addition to storing more protein and carbohydrates, pregnant mothers will experience an increase in water retention along with fat deposition in the breasts and bum. As a result of these changes, and the growth of your baby and the surrounding amniotic fluid, your weight will increase throughout pregnancy.

Changes to your musculoskeletal system occur progressively during the course of your pregnancy. As your bump grows, it will begin to place significant pressure on your core (trunk) and pelvic floor muscles. In addition, the increased weight of your bump and breasts puts stress on your spine, a subject that we will return to in the coming chapters. This increased stress is exacerbated by the elevated levels of relaxin, leading to greater joint laxity.

Managing your weight during pregnancy

Slow and steady weight gain during pregnancy is your target for you and your baby. The rate of weight gain is important, as it generally relates to the progressively increasing nutritional requirements of your baby. In addition, gradually increasing your weight is good for you, as it allows you time to adapt to your new weight and maintain an active lifestyle. And don't forget, slow, steady and appropriate weight gain will be much easier to lose post-partum. In general, your target should be for around a 14kg increase in weight across the nine months. The increase in weight is not linear, in other words you won't put on the same amount each month, as the rate of growth of your baby and related elements, such as the placenta and amniotic fluid, varies dramatically. Your weight gain should look something like the following:

- **trimester 1**: 1 to 2kg
- **trimester 2**: 7 to 8kg (up to 0.5kg per week during the fourth, fifth and sixth months)
- **trimester 3**: 3 to 4kg (no increase in weight is not uncommon in month 9 as eating becomes a struggle).

Of course, this pattern is not written in stone and you are unlikely to mirror it exactly, as it is affected by changes in your appetite and physical symptoms including nausea, reflux and heartburn. The important thing to remember is that weight gain should start slowly, increase during the second and third trimesters and slow up again prior to delivery.

> The following are guideline weight increases during pregnancy based upon the mother's pre-pregnancy body mass index (BMI):
>
> Underweight: 12.5–18kg
> Normal weight: 11.5–16kg
> Overweight: 7–11.5kg
> Obese: 5–9kg

It is important to keep a close eye on your weight. Weigh yourself weekly on the same day, at the same time of day, before eating, wearing the same clothes (naked is probably best!) and note it down. Keeping track like this will help you make better lifestyle choices and reduce the stress of worrying about your weight. Your regular health checks, which will include a weigh-in, provide a great opportunity for you to talk with your healthcare team and ensure you are on target.

Importantly, don't panic if you think you are off target. Dieting to lose weight or bingeing to increase your weight quickly is never advisable during pregnancy. Speak with your healthcare team and create a plan to return gradually to your target weight. Your weight prior to conception is important, as it will create different targets. If you are underweight when you conceive, you can gain more weight during pregnancy. In contrast, if you are overweight or obese at conception, your targets will be set at a lower level for a healthy pregnancy.

Why does it matter if I put on too much weight, or not enough weight, during pregnancy?

Putting on too much weight can have a negative effect on the development of your baby and on your own recovery post-partum.
Excessive weight can:

- make examination more difficult
- increase physical discomforts, including headaches, varicose veins and heartburn
- increase fatigue
- increase the risk of pre-term labour
- increase the risk of gestational diabetes
- increase the risk of gestational hypertension
- increase the risk of a large baby, which may result in the need for a caesarean section
- cause problems with breastfeeding
- cause problems with losing additional weight post-partum.

IMPORTANT: If you gain more than 1.5kg in a single week during the second trimester or more than 1kg in a single week in the third trimester, speak to your healthcare team.

Not putting enough weight on during pregnancy can also be problematic, potentially leading to the following problems:

- a small baby throughout pregnancy and at birth can occur, due to growth restriction in the uterus
- mothers gaining less than 9kg during pregnancy have a greater chance of a premature birth.

IMPORTANT: After the first trimester, if you fail to gain weight for more than two weeks in a row, speak with your healthcare team.

Total weight gain during pregnancy
(average increase over nine months = 14 kg)

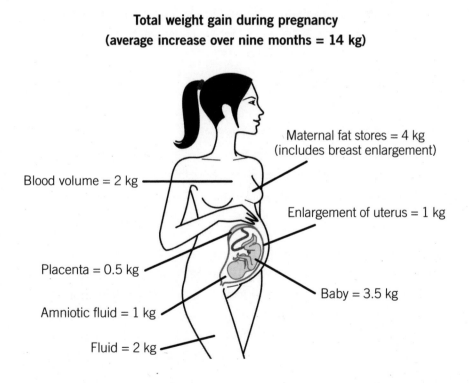

Maternal fat stores = 4 kg
(includes breast enlargement)

Blood volume = 2 kg

Enlargement of uterus = 1 kg

Placenta = 0.5 kg

Baby = 3.5 kg

Amniotic fluid = 1 kg

Fluid = 2 kg

Effects of exercise during pregnancy

Your heart rate increases as normal during exercise throughout pregnancy. Interestingly, your baby's heart rate may also rise or even lower at the same time; however, there is no lasting negative effect of this commonly observed response. Active mums-to-be have an improved cardiovascular response to exercise compared with inactive mothers. It also appears that regular exercise improves the control of blood pressure, leading to a reduced risk of gestational hypertension (high blood pressure).

Your breathing during exercise is likely to be affected while you are pregnant, particularly into the third trimester as your growing uterus pushes up on your respiratory muscles. While this makes breathing feel like harder work, it does not affect oxygen uptake, the oxygen content of your blood or oxygen supply to your baby. In fact, regular exercise helps to maintain the strength and endurance of your respiratory musculature, leading to a reduction in the symptoms of breathlessness or restriction in breathing compared to those mothers who are not physically active.

Strength exercises, including those targeting general whole-body strength, core strength and stability, and pelvic floor muscle strength, have a positive impact on your quality of life. Maintenance of whole-body strength improves your ability to cope with the activities of daily living, particularly as your weight rises. Maintenance of core strength and stability helps reduce back pain, which is reported in up to 90 per cent of pregnant women, while maintenance of pelvic floor muscle strength is something we will return to time and time again throughout this book, as it is crucial in supporting the ever-increasing weight of your uterus and helping to reduce the incidence of urinary incontinence. Furthermore, a strong, stable pelvic floor will not only help you during delivery but will help you to recover faster post-partum.

Research suggests that moderate-intensity exercise in pregnant women results in lower blood-glucose concentrations at the end of exercise. This may well be due to a reduction in the replacement of glucose into the blood rather than a greater use of glycogen. Whatever the cause, it does suggest that it may be useful, although not essential, to have healthy snacks during exercise.

Importantly, regular exercise is associated with improvements in mood and self-esteem and a reduction in depression-related symptoms, so it can have a positive effect on your mental health and quality of life throughout pregnancy and beyond.

The effects of exercise during pregnancy

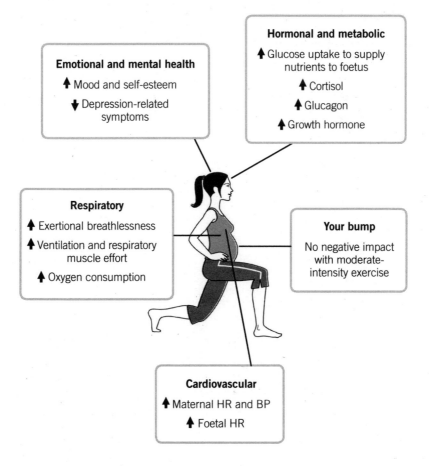

Emotional and mental health

↑ Mood and self-esteem

↓ Depression-related symptoms

Hormonal and metabolic

↑ Glucose uptake to supply nutrients to foetus

↑ Cortisol

↑ Glucagon

↑ Growth hormone

Respiratory

↑ Exertional breathlessness

↑ Ventilation and respiratory muscle effort

↑ Oxygen consumption

Your bump

No negative impact with moderate-intensity exercise

Cardiovascular

↑ Maternal HR and BP

↑ Foetal HR

In relation to your bump, there is no evidence to suggest that moderate-intensity exercise is problematic for your baby at any stage during pregnancy. In contrast to many myths that surround exercise during pregnancy, there is no effect on:

- transportation of oxygen or nutrients to your baby
- pre-term delivery in low-risk pregnancies
- birth weight in otherwise healthy mothers with an adequate energy intake.

In contrast, recent evidence suggests that women who exercise regularly throughout pregnancy have a reduced:

- incidence of gestational diabetes and hypertension
- requirement for caesarean section.

Overall, exercise that is carefully planned and controlled has a wholly positive effect on the health and well-being of you and your baby during pregnancy and should form a central part of your antenatal and post-partum care package.

Exercising safely

The contents of this book are targeted at mums-to-be with low-risk pregnancies. In general, the term 'low-risk' relates to pregnancies where there are no pre-existing health issues. This status can change throughout pregnancy and you should always seek the advice of your healthcare team before starting exercise, and regularly during the nine-month period, to ensure you are exercising safely. If your pregnancy is not considered low-risk, you can, and should, still exercise, but you will have to modify your programme. Again, speak to your healthcare team to ensure you are clear about the dos and don'ts for your particular situation.

In general, if you have been a regular exerciser prior to conception then you can continue with your exercise routine, taking into account some of the issues outlined in the following chapters. If this is not your first pregnancy, you will have some idea of what works for you and what doesn't, but it is still wise to discuss your exercise programme with your healthcare team to help them to support you as effectively as possible.

For first-time mums-to-be you should *always* speak with your healthcare team, even if you are a regular exerciser. It is important that you continually listen to your body, and adapt your exercise accordingly, throughout pregnancy. Remaining confident and positive about your exercise regime can be as important as the exercise itself!

If you have any concerns about exercise at any time during your pregnancy, you should stop and speak to your healthcare team. Below are examples of the warning signs you should look out for during exercise:

- unusual breathlessness *before* exercise
- dizziness and light-headedness
- headache (severe or prolonged)
- chest pain
- muscle weakness
- pain or swelling in calves (occurring suddenly)
- decreased foetal movement
- vaginal bleeding
- amniotic fluid leakage
- pre-term labour.

Remember, every pregnancy is different, even for existing mums. Make sure you listen to your body, and your healthcare team, to ensure you and your bump remain safe throughout pregnancy.

How hard can I exercise?

One of the most important rules of exercise during pregnancy is that you should work at, or below, moderate intensity. There are a range of ways to measure intensity during exercise, some more complex and technical than others. The most common and practical measures of exercise intensity include psychological (how you feel) and physiological (how your body is responding) factors. While there is no right or wrong way to monitor your intensity, it is important that you are able to be as accurate as possible to ensure you are not working too hard, which may mean using multiple measures to begin with until you are confident in your own ability to work to your chosen target.

Use your head

One of the simplest and most widely used psychological techniques to monitor intensity is the 'Rating of Perceived Exertion' or RPE. This approach uses your ability to detect and interpret sensations from your own body. In other words, you are monitoring how you feel and using that information to control how hard you are working.

A simple 0 to 10 scale, ranging from very easy to very hard, is used to measure your RPE. The key to the effective use of RPE is your ability to anchor the bottom (0 – 'Resting') and the top (10 – 'Maximum') of the scale. It's easiest to think of the bottom of the scale as how you feel when you are sitting watching television and the top of the scale as the hardest you have ever exercised. Having established these anchor points, you will find it much easier to set your intermediary points and, in particular, establish what moderate-intensity means for you, with an RPE of 7, which will be the primary focus of your exercise regimen throughout pregnancy.

The more you use RPE to monitor and control intensity, the easier it will become. During pregnancy, RPE is an excellent way to make sure you are working at the right intensity, as your perception of effort will naturally change as your pregnancy progresses. RPE also automatically takes into account other factors, such as the environment, to help you reduce your effort when it is hot, for example. After a while, you will not need to look at the RPE scale to know what intensity you are working at, making this the simplest of intensity-monitoring tools.

RATING OF PERCEIVED EXERTION (RPE) SCALE

1	**Resting**	Sitting down comfortably watching TV
2		
3	**Very easy**	
4	**Easy**	Able to hold a full conversation whilst exercising
5		
6	**Medium**	Able to hold a conversation in words and broken sentences whilst exercising
7		Upper limit of exercise intensity during pregnancy
8	**Hard**	Able to hold a conversation in single words whilst exercising
9		
10	**Maximum**	The hardest you have ever exercised

Use your body

Physiological measures use information from the response of your body to give you an indication of how hard you are working.

Physiological measures range in complexity (and cost!) from a simple 'Talk Test' to heart-rate monitoring.

The Talk Test is a very simple way of using your body's responses to guide you as to the intensity of exercise:

- Easy intensity: you can hold a full conversation while exercising.
- Moderate intensity: you can hold a conversation in broken sentences and words while exercising.
- Hard intensity: you can only hold a conversation in single words while exercising.

My preferred physiological measure of exercise intensity, particularly during pregnancy, is heart rate, as it takes into account all of the factors that affect how hard you are working – from your growing bump to the surrounding temperature. Importantly, your heart-rate response to exercise is specific to you, which makes it a highly effective means of controlling exercise intensity. Measuring heart-rate response to exercise is relatively simple: the harder you exercise, the higher your heart rate, and there are equally simple ways of creating your target heart-rate zones.

Before you set your target heart rates, you will need to calculate your maximum heart rate using the following simple equation:

Maximum heart rate = 220 – age

For example, to calculate the maximum heart rate of a 25-year-old mum-to-be:

Maximum heart rate = 220 – 25 = <u>195 beats per minute</u>

It is important to note that this calculation only gives a guide to your maximum heart rate. Because we use this figure to calculate your target heart rates, I suggest you use RPE (listen to your body) alongside your heart rate at the start of your exercise programme to make sure you are not working too hard.

Hitting the target

Target heart rates are based upon percentages of your maximum heart rate. During pregnancy, the key target is moderate intensity. To ensure you remain at or below this target, you should aim for an upper limit of 75 per cent of your maximum heart rate. Below is an example of how to calculate a moderate-intensity target heart rate (you can use the same equation to calculate other target heart rates by simply replacing the 75 per cent target with your chosen target).

Target heart rate = (220 – age) x 75 per cent target

For example, to calculate your moderate-intensity target heart rate (75 per cent of your maximum heart rate) as a 30-year-old mum-to-be:

Target heart rate = (220 – 30) x 0.75 = <u>142.5 beats per minute</u>

During pregnancy, it is not unusual for resting heart rate to increase. By taking account of your resting heart rate, you can improve the prediction of your target heart rate. This method uses the Karvonen equation and is a little more complex.

Target heart rate = [(220 – age – resting heart rate) x target (65, 70 or 75 per cent)] + resting heart rate

For example, to calculate your moderate-intensity target heart rate (75 per cent of your maximum heart rate) as a 35-year-old mum-to-be with a resting heart rate of 75 beats per minute:

Target heart rate = [(220 – 35 – 75) x 0.75] + 75 = <u>157.5 beats per minute</u>

Wearable tech

The easiest way to measure heart rate during exercise is to use a heart-rate monitor. There are lots of options when it comes to wearable tech, ranging from the cheap and cheerful to the expensive and highly complex. Many devices use chest straps to measure heart rate, which might be fine during the early stages of pregnancy. However, as your bump and breasts grow, and your skin becomes more sensitive, it is advisable to invest in a monitor that measures your heart rate at the wrist. There are a number of options but devices such as a Fitbit will not only measure your heart rate during exercise but also provide you with a whole host of other data – from your step and calorie count to the length and quality of your sleep. You can also create a community and share your data with antenatal friends, your healthcare team, etc.

> **Top Tip:** The Talk Test is a great way to estimate how hard you are working. In general, during easy exercise (i.e. an RPE of 3 to 5) you are able to hold a full conversation without breaks. As the exercise moves into the moderate territory (i.e. an RPE of 5 to 7), your conversation will be broken as your breathing rate increases, and while you will be able to talk, you won't be able to sing (which might already be true before starting exercise!). During high-intensity exercise (i.e. an RPE of 8 to 10), you can only speak in short sentences or single words. So if you're unsure whether you've hit an RPE of 7 or not, have a chat!

Variety is the spice of life!

You don't have to complete all of your exercise sessions in one go. Whether it's 30 minutes of aerobic exercise, a strength or core strength and stability session, you can break them up into smaller, more manageable chunks. For example, instead of your 30-minute aerobic session you can gain the same benefits from three 10-minute sessions spread across the day. Equally, you can choose to complete just one set of strength or core strength and stability exercises and pick up the other sets later in the day.

In addition to changing the duration of sessions, for aerobic exercise you could vary the intensity by using an interval or fartlek structure. Interval exercise is where you divide your workout into periods of moderate-intensity (RPE of 7, or 75 per cent of your maximum heart rate) activity interspersed with periods of rest. For example, ten 2-minute bouts at a moderate intensity with a 1-minute rest between each 2-minute bout. Alternatively, you could try fartlek (meaning speed play), where you change the intensity of exercise from easy to moderate throughout your workout. For example, you could try 2 minutes at an RPE of 4 or 5, followed by 1 minute at an RPE of 7, repeated 10 times. Fartlek can add variety to your session, which helps maintain your motivation to exercise.

For aerobic exercise, it's also worth considering trying different types of exercise. Don't limit yourself to one thing. By mixing up your sessions, you'll ensure you maintain your enjoyment and motivation. And don't discount a new exercise that you haven't tried before; learning a new skill, something we call 'mastering', is a proven way to enhance your motivation. Of course, make sure you seek expert advice from a qualified trainer before trying out anything new. Going along to a prenatal class or one led by a qualified instructor is the simplest and safest way to broaden your exercise menu. (Please see the exercise cycle chart on page 115.)

It's all in your mind! Exercise results in the release of endorphins, which are sometimes called the 'happy hormones'. It is common to experience a high following exercise, as the release of endorphins makes you feel energized and positive. Remember, you don't have to be an athlete to benefit from the positive effect of endorphins; any exercise will leave you feeling great.

The expectant dad

Pregnancy is not just about mum (although most of it is!). 'You're going to be a dad!' is one of the most exciting announcements a man is ever likely to hear, but the pregnancy journey can be packed with trepidation and leave the father feeling utterly superfluous as a side-line observer while the events of the next nine months unfold.

But providing your sperm for the creation of life is far from the end of your responsibilities. Fatherhood, much like motherhood, begins before conception and continues throughout pregnancy and beyond. We have already discussed the role of a healthy lifestyle in improving paternal fertility and here we shall discuss its importance in helping you to support your partner through the next nine months. Your quality of life directly impacts on your partner and your unborn baby. So making the right lifestyle choices and working with your partner to achieve and maintain the right exercise regime, diet and lifestyle will be central to a successful pregnancy and birth.

Good communication and understanding are vital to helping you support your partner over the next nine months. Being able to talk openly will allow you to gain a better understanding of how she is feeling, both physically and emotionally, and help you to offer the appropriate encouragement or reassurance. It's also important to remember that your own fears about pregnancy and becoming a dad can lead to anxiety and stress that you may project on to your partner. So good communication can help to reduce the stress of pregnancy for both of you.

Don't assume that knowing about pregnancy is just for girls! Do some research of your own and find out about pregnancy and the changes your partner is experiencing. Try to attend antenatal classes. In particular, father-only classes can be an incredibly helpful place for you to share your concerns and fears as well as learning about various coping strategies for you and your partner as you journey through the next nine months together. And importantly, don't be a man about it! Speak to friends who are also expecting or are already dads; a worry shared is a worry halved. There are some excellent books on fatherhood that can provide detailed insight into all aspects of pregnancy for expectant dads. So don't be a spectator, be part of the team.

As a dad, you should also be supporting your partner by adopting the same healthy lifestyle choices that she is being encouraged to make. It's not rocket science but sometimes dads-to-be can forget what an impact their unhealthy habits can have on their partner. So you should:

- Definitely stop smoking (a piece of advice that I would give whether you are a father-to-be or not!). Passive smoking has a harmful effect on your partner and your baby.
- Moderate your alcohol consumption. Think about your partner: there's nothing worse than watching someone else have a nice glass of wine when you're abstaining.
- Eat healthily. The recipe suggestions in this book are not just for expectant mums; when you sit down for meals together, think about eating the same food as your partner.
- Be an exercise buddy. You don't have to do every session together but joining them for a walk or a regular workout can provide motivation and support, and gives you an opportunity to chat in a different environment.
- Become part of the pregnancy team! Rather than sitting on the sidelines, you can exercise with your partner, making you a more valuable team member and optimizing the chances of you and your partner having a healthy, relaxed and more enjoyable pregnancy.

FAQs

What happens to my metabolism during pregnancy?

Pregnancy leads to an increase in your metabolic rate of up to 25 per cent, peaking towards the end of your second trimester and remaining elevated until delivery. This is accompanied by an increase in heart rate as you pump more blood around your body (termed your 'cardiac output'). In addition, your breathing rate increases to accommodate the increased energy and oxygen demands of your developing baby.

How much more energy do I need to consume during pregnancy?

From the start of trimester 2 (after 13 weeks), you will require around an extra 300Kcals per day to meet the increased metabolic needs of pregnancy. Of course, exercise on top of being pregnant adds an extra calorie requirement. The amount of energy required will depend on how often, how hard and for how long you exercise. The increasing weight of your baby will also add to the energy demands as you move towards delivery. The best way to keep an eye on your energy intake is to track your weight gain during pregnancy and check you are on target (see pages 20–1).

Do I need more carbohydrates during pregnancy?

During pregnancy, you will use carbohydrate at a greater rate, both at rest and during exercise, compared to when you're not pregnant. So a little extra carbohydrate in your diet won't hurt but remember we are talking about complex carbohydrates such as potatoes, pasta, rice, etc., not sugars, which can be problematic in excess.

Is it safe to do exercise classes while I'm pregnant?

It really depends on the type of class and what stage of pregnancy you are at. During the first trimester, if you are having a normal pregnancy, you can continue to exercise as normal with no real exclusions. As you move through the second trimester into the third, the additional weight you begin to carry will affect how you move and also particular areas of the body such as your pelvic floor. As this progresses, you will need to reduce the intensity of your exercise and, more importantly, think carefully about impact exercises, i.e. aerobics, CrossFit, step, etc.

Will my baby be born early if I exercise during pregnancy?

Research suggests that for otherwise healthy mothers with low-risk pregnancies moderate-intensity exercise has no impact on gestational age. For higher-risk pregnancies, you should always seek the advice of your healthcare team.

Can I drink alcohol while I'm pregnant?

This is a difficult question to answer with absolute certainty and the simplest solution is not to drink at all. If this is difficult to achieve, then it is clear that you should not exceed one to two units of alcohol (half to a pint of lager, one to two single shots, or a small glass of wine) one to two times per week. (For further advice, check out the NHS website: http://www.nhs.uk/Conditions/pregnancy-and-baby/pages/alcohol-medicines-drugs-pregnant.aspx). My advice is to stop, or reduce your alcohol consumption to an absolute minimum, to ensure you limit any negative impact on your developing baby. Importantly, alcohol can affect the development of your baby's brain, so think about my mantra when you feel like a drink: abstinence makes the brain go stronger!

Can I run during pregnancy?

The simple answer to this question is yes; however, there are important caveats, along with a host of guidelines, if you wish to continue (or start) running during pregnancy. Overleaf is a table to help guide you through your decision.

RUNNING DURING PREGNANCY

	Can I run?	How should I structure my running? How long can I run for and at what intensity?	Should I be doing anything else to support my running?
Never run before	There is no reason why you cannot start running; however, alternative forms of exercise might be better for you. Importantly, it is inadvisable to start running in trimesters 2 or 3.	Start with walking and introduce short episodes of jogging interspersed with walking or recovery. Build up gradually. Thirty minutes should be your maximum duration. Consider moving to fartlek or interval running in trimester 2 and stopping in trimester 3. Do not exceed an RPE of 7 (75 per cent of your maximum heart rate). **Listen carefully to your body.**	• Core strength and stability • Pelvic floor exercises • Run on flat, even surfaces • Take care not to overheat • Always carry fluid with you
Infrequent runner	As you have run before conception, you can continue running. However, as you are unlikely to be fully conditioned to running, you should take extra care to control intensity in trimester 2. It may be advisable to choose a different activity in trimester 3.	Continue with your running from pre-conception; however, consider reducing the duration (maximum of 30 minutes) and ensure you do not exceed an RPE of 7 (75 per cent of your maximum heart rate). Consider moving to fartlek or interval running in trimester 2 and stopping in trimester 3. **Listen carefully to your body.**	• Core strength and stability • Pelvic floor exercises • Run on flat, even surfaces • Take care not to overheat • Always carry fluid with you
Regular runner	As a regular runner, you will be fully conditioned for running across all three trimesters if you are able to maintain your regular routine. Listen to your body as you progress, particularly	Continue your running from pre-conception. If there are no breaks in your routine (for example due to morning sickness, etc.), you can continue running throughout your pregnancy. If you have to stop running or encounter problems running as your	• Core strength and stability • Pelvic floor exercises • Run on flat, even surfaces • Take care not to overheat

	Can I run?	How should I structure my running? How long can I run for and at what intensity?	Should I be doing anything else to support my running?
	into trimester 3, and reduce/stop running if necessary.	bump grows, consider fartlek or interval running. Longer runs are not a problem as long as you do not overheat, and avoid dehydration and low energy levels. Do not exceed an RPE of 7 (75 per cent of your maximum heart rate). **Listen carefully to your body.**	• Always carry fluid with you • Consider carrying snacks for longer runs
Competitive runner	You should be able to run throughout your pregnancy if you are able to maintain your level of conditioning. As a competitive athlete, you must pay careful attention to intensity (don't push too hard). With the increased weight and change in your centre of gravity in trimester 3, think carefully about your and your baby's health; remember that you will be able to return to running post-partum.	Continue your running from pre-conception. If there are no breaks in your running (for example due to morning sickness, etc.), you can continue running throughout your pregnancy. If you have to stop running or encounter problems running as your bump grows, consider fartlek or interval running. Longer runs are not a problem as long as you do not overheat, and avoid dehydration and low energy levels. Evidence suggests intensities of up to 81 per cent of your maximum heart rate are not problematic – listen to your body and be very careful not to overheat if you do move up to this intensity. **Listen carefully to your body.**	• Core strength and stability • Pelvic floor exercises • Run on flat, even surfaces • Take care not to overheat • Always carry fluid with you • Consider carrying snacks for longer runs

PREGNANCY TRIVIA

DO NOT SMOKE!

Cigarette smoke contains more than 4,000 chemicals that travel from your lungs into your bloodstream through your placenta and umbilical cord, directly to your baby. In addition to the damaging effect of these chemicals, the oxygen supply to your baby will also be reduced. These effects last for up to 15 minutes following each cigarette!

High intensity

In general, high-intensity exercise is not advised at any stage during pregnancy. However, for those mums-to-be who were highly fit prior to becoming pregnant, research suggests that exercise intensities of up to 81 per cent of your maximum heart rate do not lead to significant adverse effects for mother or baby.

Water, water everywhere!

One litre of water weighs 1kg. By weighing yourself before and after exercise you can calculate how much fluid you have lost and replace it with an appropriate-size drink.

Weighing in

Gaining excessive amounts of weight during pregnancy increases the incidence of hypertension (high blood pressure), gestational diabetes and foetal macrosomia (high birth weight above 8lb 13oz; however, complications are greater at weights above 9lb 15oz), which impact on the health of your baby during pregnancy and into their future lives. Exercise and diet are the cornerstones of reaching and maintaining a healthy weight.

My legs look like a road map!

It is not uncommon to suffer from varicose veins during pregnancy. Physical and hormonal changes during pregnancy can result in the failure of the valves inside your veins, leading to the pooling of blood. This pooling creates the characteristic large bluish veins, particularly on the back of the legs. Regular exercise can reduce the development of varicose veins and you can also follow these simple tips: avoid standing or sitting in one position for too long, avoid crossing your legs and avoid excessive weight gain.

Olympic pregnancy

A host of pregnant athletes have competed at the Olympic Games and even won medals but the gold medal goes to Nur Suryani Mohamed Taibi, who became the most pregnant Olympic athlete in history when she competed in rifle shooting while eight months pregnant at the 2012 Games!

3

The First Trimester:
Months 1 to 3

You and your bump

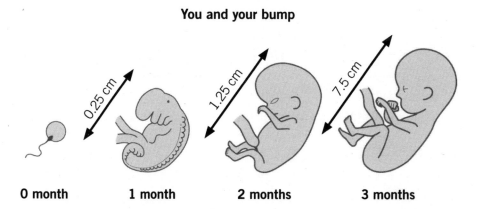

| 0 month | 1 month | 2 months | 3 months |

In the first month (weeks 1 to 4) of pregnancy, there are many amazing things going on inside you and, while your bump is yet to show itself to others, you will start to experience a range of early pregnancy symptoms that are driven by changing hormone levels. Given the lack of any physical changes in these early weeks, you would not be alone in passing off these symptoms as something other than pregnancy even if, inside you, the amazing cycle of creation has begun.

Your pregnancy is given a start date of the first day of your last period. So for the first two weeks you're not actually pregnant. But following ovulation (around two weeks after the first day of your last period), when the egg is fertilized by the strongest of your partner's little swimmers, you're on your way. Once fertilized, the division of cells begins, with the original single-celled zygote rapidly changing into a tiny ball of cells (called a blastocyst if you're interested!) that travels down your fallopian tube, transforming into an embryo as it journeys along its path towards your uterus, where, at around week 4, it will embed itself. At this point, a major division takes place: a portion of the cells will become your baby and the other portion will become his or her placenta, which acts as the link to its life-support system – you! At the same time, the amniotic sac and yolk sac begin to form. By the end of week 4, an amazing transformation has taken place from egg and sperm to an embryo that has already begun to grow into three specialist layers that will become the incredibly complex body parts from brain to skin.

During the second month (weeks 5 to 8), your baby grows from the size of an orange pip to the size of a grape – 1.25cm in length (measured from head to toe). This month sees the growth of the first vital system – the cardiovascular system – the health of which will be of key importance throughout the life of this new being. The heart, which starts out as two small heart tubes, begins to beat at around 80 beats per minute; this will increase to around 150 beats per minute by the time the month is up.

In week 6, your baby starts to develop the neural tube that will carry the spinal cord, along with the beginnings of the jaw, cheeks, chin, nose, eyes and ears.

In week 7, new brain cells are being developed at an astonishing rate (around 100 cells per minute!). The buds that grow into arms and legs start to develop – two into hands, arms and shoulders, and two into feet, legs and hips.

By the end of month 2, the embryo that resembled a tadpole is beginning to look more like a baby as the facial features continue to develop along with the arms and legs. Even at this early stage your baby will begin to move, with tiny twitches of its back and limbs. Although you won't be able to feel any of these tiny movements, it is likely you will experience a range of physical and emotional changes that may affect you in a variety of ways (see table overleaf).

Your baby's movements will continue to increase over the next five weeks, with the development of muscles as he or she grows rapidly, more than quadrupling in size to around 7.5cm (the size of a tangerine) by the end of the first trimester. But it is still too early to feel these movements; that will begin in the second trimester. Along with the muscles, the bones and cartilage are beginning to form. Organs are developing, including the kidneys, which are now producing urine.

By the end of week 11, the ovaries in girls and the testes in boys are in the process of developing.

By week 13, the foetus will look much more like a baby, with individual fingers and toes, a face, including ears, open nasal passages and a mouth with a tongue and a palate.

The end of trimester 1 marks the point at which your baby moves from embryo to foetus. At this point, your baby will only weigh around 25g but you can expect an increase in your weight of around 1 to 2kg. The overall increase in your weight is primarily associated with the forming of the placenta and amniotic fluid, the enlarged uterus and breasts, and increased adipose (fat) stores – all in preparation for the months ahead.

What changes can I expect in the first trimester of pregnancy?

Increases in a number of hormones including oestrogen, progesterone and human chorionic gonadotropin (HCG) may lead to a range of physical and emotional changes; the individual nature of pregnancy means that you may experience none or all of these. Indeed, you may have other less common symptoms that are not reported in books, magazines or online. It is important to remember that if you have any concerns at all you should speak with your healthcare professional.

The following are common changes you may experience.

PHYSICAL AND EMOTIONAL CHANGES: TRIMESTER 1

	Month 1	Month 2	Month 3
PHYSICAL			
Fatigue: it's not unusual to lack energy and feel more sleepy than usual	✓	✓	✓
Nausea (with or without vomiting)	✓	✓	✓ inc. excessive saliva
Bloating, flatulence and urinating more often (as the increasing size of the uterus presses down on your bladder)	✓	✓	✓
Indigestion, heartburn, reflux		✓	✓
Constipation		✓	
Breast changes, including weight, size, tenderness, tingling, and darkening of the areolas	✓	✓ inc. blue veins under the skin	✓ inc. blue veins under the skin
Veins under the skin of the stomach and legs			✓
Occasional headaches		✓	✓
Occasional dizziness and light-headedness		✓	✓
Food fetishes or dislikes		✓	✓
Increased appetite			✓

	Month 1	Month 2	Month 3
Spotting or staining is possible, associated with implantation of the embryo (usually around 5 to 10 days after conception, with around a third of women experiencing 'implantation bleeding')	✓		
Vaginal discharge (white in colour)		✓	✓
Growth of your bump		✓	✓
EMOTIONAL			
Mood swings, irritability, irrationality, unexpected crying (heightened premenstrual syndrome)	✓	✓	✓

Exercise and the first trimester

In general, you can continue your normal exercise programme throughout the first trimester. Inside your uterus, the foetus is so small at this stage that it is well protected in your abdominal cavity. Even traditional sit-up type exercises, running and weightlifting are possible during the first trimester. There are, of course, a number of caveats to this advice, which include the following:

- This general advice is specifically for low-risk pregnancies. If you have a higher-risk pregnancy, speak with your healthcare team before embarking on an exercise programme.
- What you are able to do is directly related to what you were doing *prior* to becoming pregnant and your level of conditioning.

If you are starting to exercise for the first time (or after a long period of time without exercising), you will need to progress slowly. A good tip is to think about starting with trimester 2 exercises (see Chapter 4).

- Be careful not to overheat (see below).

- Keep the exercise intensity below an RPE (Rating of Perceived Exertion is a measure of how hard you feel you are working) of 7, or 75 per cent of your maximum heart rate (see Chapter 2).

- It is advisable to avoid contact sports or activities that have the potential for impact injuries.

- Listen to your body. Common sense should always prevail, so you should never push yourself beyond where you feel comfortable and stop immediately if you have any concerns or discomfort.

Heating up

During pregnancy, your metabolism (the amount of energy you pro-duce and consume) speeds up in relation to the increased energy demand from supporting your developing baby and the host of other changes taking place in your body, from greater red blood cell produc-tion to the enlargement of your breasts. All of this takes energy and therefore leads to an increase in what is termed 'Resting Metabolic Rate' (RMR). This increased metabolic rate due to pregnancy, com-bined with a metabolic rise induced by exercise, leads to the heating-up of your body. In response, the body steps up its attempts to get rid of this heat by increasing the sweat rate and diverting blood flow to the skin (which is what makes you look like a sweaty tomato!). Impor-tantly, sweating can lead to dehydration, which is why you should always make sure you take in plenty of fluids during your workout.

The amount of heat you generate is directly related to the intensity of exercise (how hard you are working): the harder you work, the hotter you get. In addition, the environment you are exercising in can make a big difference: the hotter and/or more humid the environment, the more you heat up. Why does it matter? There is limited research on this topic but the general consensus is that you should avoid becoming excessively hot during exercise. This is particularly important during the first trimester, as it is one of the most sensitive periods for your developing foetus.

Measuring how hot you get during exercise is very difficult to do, so here are a few tips to guide you:

- **Moderation:** avoid exercising too intensely in order not to generate a lot of heat. Exercise up to an RPE of 7, or a heart rate below 75 per cent of maximum. At this intensity, your body will be able to manage the increased heat and hold your core (body) temperature stable.

- **Fluid:** sweating can lead to dehydration, so make sure you have a drink with you during exercise and take a sip regularly. Water is fine, as you won't be exercising for prolonged periods. Limit your use of carbohydrate/sports drinks, as they can add significant calories to your diet without you realizing.

- **Go easy in the heat:** make sure you take into account the environment. If exercising in a confined space without adequate ventilation, or if it is hot and/or humid, reduce the intensity a little to compensate.

- **Clothing:** always wear appropriate clothing for the activity and the environment. Think about layers that you can remove as you begin to warm up during exercise and which you can put back on when you've finished.

Warm–up and cool–down

Never start an exercise session, including aerobic exercise, without a warm-up, progressively increasing in intensity up to the intended level for your session, and some flexibility exercises. The purpose of a warm-up is to get your body (and mind) ready for exercise by gradually:

- increasing heart rate and therefore blood flow
- redistributing blood to the working muscles
- increasing ventilation (breathing)
- increasing the temperature of your muscles
- increasing your range of motion.

A warm-up will improve your performance, reduce the potential for injury and thus protect your baby. In addition to warming up, don't stop exercise abruptly; cooling down is equally important, as it will:

- bring your metabolism back down to near resting levels
- redistribute your blood away from your muscles
- reduce your core and muscle temperature.

On the following pages is an example of both an aerobic and flexibility warm-up/cool-down you can use throughout your pregnancy. By using music, you can set the pace of your warm-up/cool-down – perhaps choosing an increasing tempo during your warm-up and a decreasing tempo during your cool-down.

AEROBIC WARM-UP: TRIMESTER 1

Repeat each of the exercises for 30 seconds to a minute.

Use music to dictate timing. Choose a tempo of music that you can maintain without excessive fatigue (an RPE of 7 or less, or 75 per cent or less of your maximum heart rate; see Chapter 2).

Remember, it is very important to maintain good posture throughout each exercise: draw your shoulder blades back, stand tall through your spine, draw your abdominals in slightly and tuck your pelvis under (bring your pubic bone up towards your belly button).

1 Marching

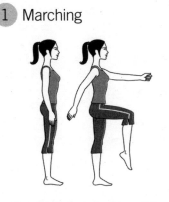

- Stand with feet shoulder-width apart with soft knees
- Draw your belly button towards your back and tighten your bum and thighs
- Lift your right knee up as high as is comfortable (maintain balance) while swinging your left arm forward
- Return to start position under control
- Repeat for your left knee

2 Side step

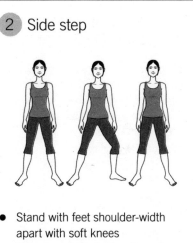

- Stand with feet shoulder-width apart with soft knees
- Draw your belly button towards your back and tighten your bum and thighs
- Step to the right with your right foot and then your left
- Step to the left (back to start position) with your left foot then your right

3 Toe tap

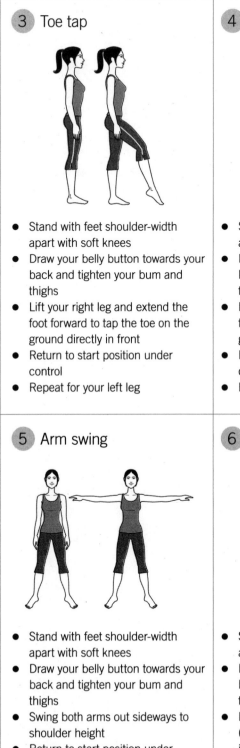

- Stand with feet shoulder-width apart with soft knees
- Draw your belly button towards your back and tighten your bum and thighs
- Lift your right leg and extend the foot forward to tap the toe on the ground directly in front
- Return to start position under control
- Repeat for your left leg

4 Heel tap

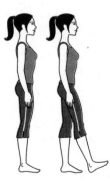

- Stand with feet shoulder-width apart with soft knees
- Draw your belly button towards your back and tighten your bum and thighs
- Lift your right leg and extend the foot forward to tap the heel on the ground directly in front
- Return to start position under control
- Repeat for your left leg

5 Arm swing

- Stand with feet shoulder-width apart with soft knees
- Draw your belly button towards your back and tighten your bum and thighs
- Swing both arms out sideways to shoulder height
- Return to start position under control

6 Squat

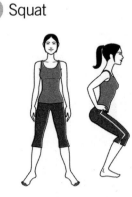

- Stand with feet shoulder-width apart with soft knees
- Draw your belly button towards your back and tighten your bum and thighs
- Bend both legs to a maximum of 90° (use a chair to touch your bottom on if you're unsure where to stop)
- Return to start position under control

Knee lift

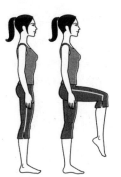

- Stand with feet shoulder-width apart with soft knees
- Draw your belly button towards your back and tighten your bum and thighs
- Lift your right knee up as high as is comfortable (maintain balance)
- Return to start position under control
- Repeat for your left knee

8 Feet to bum

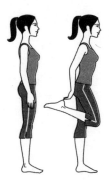

- Stand with feet shoulder-width apart with soft knees
- Draw your belly button towards your back and tighten your bum and thighs
- Lift your right heel up to touch your bottom
- Return to start position under control
- Repeat for your left heel

9 Side swing

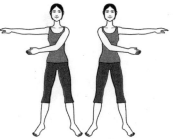

- Stand with feet shoulder-width apart with soft knees
- Draw your belly button towards your back and tighten your bum and thighs
- Swing both arms towards the right
- Return to start position under control
- Repeat to the left

10 Sumo squat

- Stand with feet wider than shoulder-width apart (as wide as you feel comfortable) with soft knees
- Draw your belly button towards your back and tighten your bum and thighs
- Bend both legs to a maximum of 90° (use a chair to touch your bottom on if you're unsure where to stop)
- Return to start position under control

FLEXIBILITY: TRIMESTER 1

While completing these exercises, it is important not to over-stretch. With the rise in levels of circulating relaxin leading to increased joint laxity, make sure you maintain a safe level of stretch.

Also remember to maintain good posture throughout each exercise whether standing or sitting.

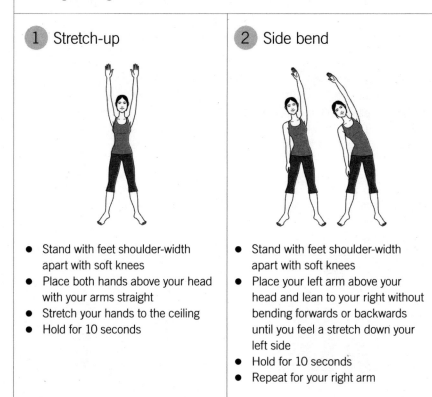

1 Stretch-up

- Stand with feet shoulder-width apart with soft knees
- Place both hands above your head with your arms straight
- Stretch your hands to the ceiling
- Hold for 10 seconds

2 Side bend

- Stand with feet shoulder-width apart with soft knees
- Place your left arm above your head and lean to your right without bending forwards or backwards until you feel a stretch down your left side
- Hold for 10 seconds
- Repeat for your right arm

3 Triceps stretch

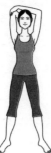

- Stand with feet shoulder-width apart with soft knees
- Lift your right arm above your head and bend it at the elbow, with the hand pointing down your back
- Cup the elbow with the opposite hand and ease the elbow towards your head until you feel a stretch in the back of the upper arm
- Hold for 10 seconds
- Repeat for your left arm

4 Upper back

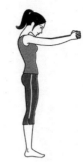

- Stand with feet shoulder-width apart with soft knees
- Interlock your fingers and stretch your arms out in front of you with palms facing inwards
- Round your shoulders, push out your shoulder blades and stretch your hands forwards
- Hold for 10 seconds

5 Chest

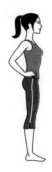

- Stand with feet shoulder-width apart with soft knees
- Place your hands on your hips
- Pull your elbows backwards and push your chest out until you feel a stretch across your chest
- Hold for 10 seconds

6 Shoulder

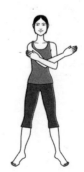

- Stand with feet shoulder-width apart with soft knees
- Bring your right arm across your chest towards the opposite shoulder without rotating the upper body
- Cup the upper arm with your hand and pull the arm towards your chest until you feel a stretch in the back of your shoulder
- Hold for 10 seconds
- Repeat for your left arm

7 Shoulder roll

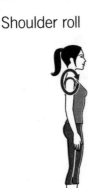

- Stand with feet shoulder-width apart with soft knees
- Without swinging your arms, rotate your shoulders forwards
- Repeat 10 times
- Repeat, rotating your shoulders backwards

8 Side lunge

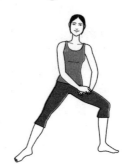

- Stand with feet slightly more than shoulder-width apart
- Looking forwards, keep your body upright
- Keeping your right leg straight, bend your left leg until you feel a stretch in the inner right thigh
- Hold for 10 seconds
- Repeat for your right leg

9 Quads

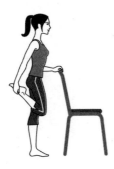

- Stand upright and stable
- Bend your right knee and pull the heel to your bum (hold on to something for stability if required)
- Hold the ankle of the bent leg and pull the foot into your bum without leaning forwards (keep a straight line between shoulder, hip and knee)
- Hold for 10 seconds
- Repeat for your left leg

10 Hamstring

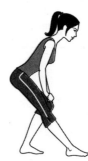

- Stand with feet shoulder-width apart with soft knees
- Take a step forwards with your right leg
- Bend the back leg, keeping the front leg straight
- Bend forwards and pull your toes towards you until you feel a stretch along the back of your thigh
- Hold for 10 seconds
- Repeat for your left leg

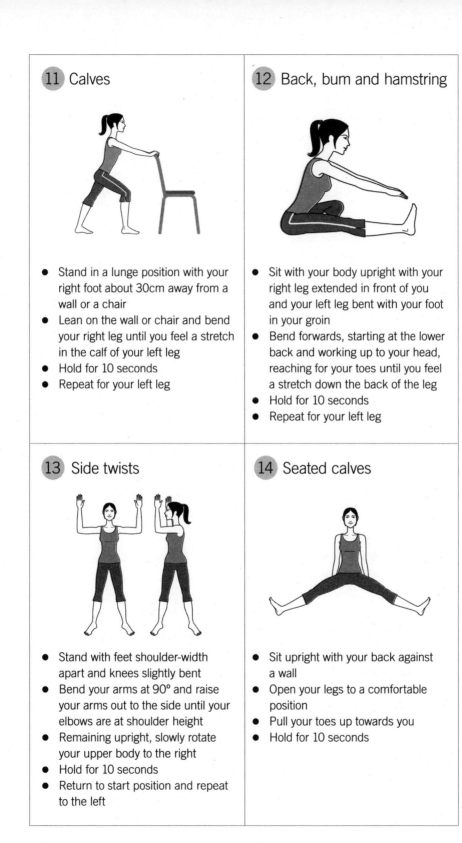

11 Calves

- Stand in a lunge position with your right foot about 30cm away from a wall or a chair
- Lean on the wall or chair and bend your right leg until you feel a stretch in the calf of your left leg
- Hold for 10 seconds
- Repeat for your left leg

12 Back, bum and hamstring

- Sit with your body upright with your right leg extended in front of you and your left leg bent with your foot in your groin
- Bend forwards, starting at the lower back and working up to your head, reaching for your toes until you feel a stretch down the back of the leg
- Hold for 10 seconds
- Repeat for your left leg

13 Side twists

- Stand with feet shoulder-width apart and knees slightly bent
- Bend your arms at 90° and raise your arms out to the side until your elbows are at shoulder height
- Remaining upright, slowly rotate your upper body to the right
- Hold for 10 seconds
- Return to start position and repeat to the left

14 Seated calves

- Sit upright with your back against a wall
- Open your legs to a comfortable position
- Pull your toes up towards you
- Hold for 10 seconds

Aerobic exercise

During the first trimester, you have almost free rein to choose any type of aerobic exercise from walking to swimming, and cycling to rowing; even running is acceptable during the first trimester, and beyond if you were a regular runner before you became pregnant. There are some activities that, while not forbidden, do carry additional risk, for example scuba diving, because of the impact of increased pressure on your blood pressure and volume, and skiing, because of the chances of an impact injury to you and your baby. You should assess the risk of these types of activities and decide whether you are comfortable to continue. If in doubt, seek professional advice.

You can also keep up with your regular exercise classes as long as you follow the same general advice for all aerobic activities (see above and page 49). A class of about 30 to 45 minutes should be fine but remember that it is common for classes to be of high intensity and to take place in hot, humid environments. This shouldn't stop you from making classes part of your weekly routine but do remember to keep the intensity at moderate levels, wear appropriate clothing to avoid overheating and make sure you have a drink with you.

The recommended levels of aerobic activity for health are 30 minutes per day of moderate-intensity exercise at least 5 days per week. You can follow the same guideline during this stage of your pregnancy – perhaps aiming for five aerobic sessions per week if that is what you feel comfortable doing. However, as a general rule of thumb, the lower the intensity, the longer you will be able to exercise. So if you are walking, there is no reason why you cannot go beyond 30 minutes. In addition to the general advice, the main thing to think about when you go for longer durations (over 60 minutes) is your nutrition; make sure you keep your energy and hydration levels topped up by having adequate amounts of healthy snacks and drinks with you.

Aerobic exercises that are safe during trimester 1:

- walking
- running (particularly if you are already a runner)
- cross-trainer
- stepper
- rowing ergometer
- cycling (stationary/gym bikes are less risky but outdoor cycling is OK)
- recumbent cycling
- versa climber
- arm ergometer
- swimming

Strength exercise

Resistance exercise, whether in the gym using machines or at home using free weights, is an important part of your exercise programme. Maintaining muscle strength will improve your ability to cope with daily life and the anatomical changes that take place as your baby grows. Much the same as with aerobic exercise, during trimester 1 you have free rein over what type of strength exercise you choose. Again, it will very much depend on your exercise programme prior to becoming pregnant. If you have not undertaken strength exercises before, or it's been a long time since you lifted a weight, make sure you start very light, preferably with no additional weight (just using your own body weight), and increase gradually. Importantly, if you intend to incorporate machine weights into your routine but have never used them before, make sure you speak with an exercise professional to seek advice on the correct techniques to employ.

In general, you should aim to lift low weights with higher repetition. You can progressively increase the number of repetitions to improve your strength, but ensure you maintain the correct techniques to avoid injury. Below is an example programme for strength that you can use throughout trimester 1.

STRENGTH AND TONE: TRIMESTER 1

For these exercises, you should select a weight with which you can complete all the repetitions of each exercise (and that can mean no weight at all). The weight you choose is likely to be different for each exercise; however, you can use the same weight and increase the number of repetitions if you feel the weight is too light. Alternatively, you should consider increasing the weight of your dumbbells when you can easily complete all repetitions.

Always complete the exercises slowly and under control. Rest for around 1 minute between exercises. Remember to keep your RPE at 7 or below, avoid overheating and have fluid with you to drink when required.

1 Squat

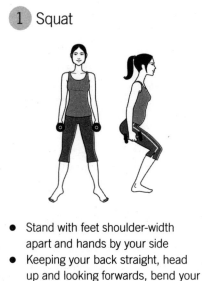

- Stand with feet shoulder-width apart and hands by your side
- Keeping your back straight, head up and looking forwards, bend your legs to 90°
- Return to start position and repeat 20 times

2 Upright row

- Stand with feet shoulder-width apart, your arms straight, palms facing towards your thighs
- Bending both arms, bring your hands upwards until they reach the level of your shoulders
- Return to start position and repeat 20 times

3 Sumo squat

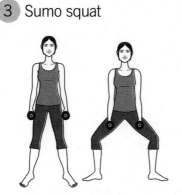

- Stand with feet wider than shoulder-width apart (as wide as you feel comfortable) with soft knees
- Keeping your back straight, head up and looking forwards, bend both legs to a maximum of 90° (use a chair to touch your bottom on if you're unsure where to stop)
- Return to start position under control and repeat 20 times

4 Side arm lift

- Stand with feet shoulder-width apart and palms facing the side of your thighs
- Keep your back straight, head up and look forwards
- Keeping your arms straight, raise both arms directly to your side until they are level with your shoulders
- Return to start position and repeat 20 times

5 Lunge

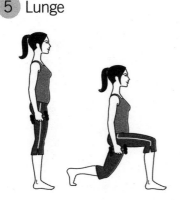

- Stand with feet shoulder-width apart
- Keeping your upper body upright and looking forwards, take a large step forwards with your right foot and bend your front leg to 90°, keeping your knee over your foot
- Return to start position and repeat for your left leg
- Repeat 10 times

6 Shoulder press

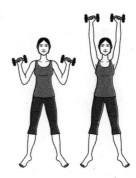

- Stand with feet shoulder-width apart
- Bring your hands to your shoulders with your elbows down
- Extend both arms upwards above your head until they are straight
- Return to start position and repeat 20 times

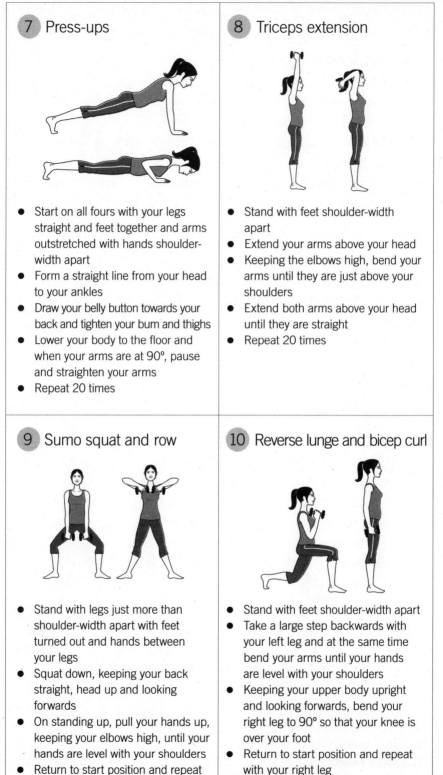

7 Press-ups

- Start on all fours with your legs straight and feet together and arms outstretched with hands shoulder-width apart
- Form a straight line from your head to your ankles
- Draw your belly button towards your back and tighten your bum and thighs
- Lower your body to the floor and when your arms are at 90°, pause and straighten your arms
- Repeat 20 times

8 Triceps extension

- Stand with feet shoulder-width apart
- Extend your arms above your head
- Keeping the elbows high, bend your arms until they are just above your shoulders
- Extend both arms above your head until they are straight
- Repeat 20 times

9 Sumo squat and row

- Stand with legs just more than shoulder-width apart with feet turned out and hands between your legs
- Squat down, keeping your back straight, head up and looking forwards
- On standing up, pull your hands up, keeping your elbows high, until your hands are level with your shoulders
- Return to start position and repeat 20 times

10 Reverse lunge and bicep curl

- Stand with feet shoulder-width apart
- Take a large step backwards with your left leg and at the same time bend your arms until your hands are level with your shoulders
- Keeping your upper body upright and looking forwards, bend your right leg to 90° so that your knee is over your foot
- Return to start position and repeat with your right leg
- Repeat 10 times

The abdominal muscles

Your growing baby sits inside your abdominal cavity and as he or she grows they begin to increase the pressure on the muscles that span the abdominal cavity from the ribs to the pelvis. The muscles particularly at risk due to your ever-increasing bump are the *rectus abdominis* (commonly called the 'abdominals' or 'abs'), which are positioned down the front of your abdomen. The abdominals are two parallel muscles, separated by a midline band of connective tissue called the *linea alba*. Three bands of connective tissue running horizontally across the abdominals subdivide them into eight muscle bellies that create the characteristic 'six pack' (some people have an 'eight pack'!). As your baby grows (along with the expansion of your uterus due to the increasing size of the placenta and volume of amniotic fluid), the abdominal muscles are stretched, placing stress on the *linea alba*. Alongside the increased stress, the release of the hormone relaxin (see Chapter 2) leads to a stretching of the *linea alba*. Eventually, the *linea alba* may split (termed '*diastasis recti*'), commonly starting at the belly button. This split can travel up or down but either way it results in weakened abdominals, which in turn may place additional stress on your back. For this reason, it is important that you maintain your core strength (the other muscles supporting your back) to avoid chronic back pain.

During the first trimester, you are unlikely to experience any issues with your abdominal muscles, as the growth of the foetus does not cause significant enlargement of your uterus. However, it is important to maintain the condition of your abdominals and core muscles throughout the first trimester to ensure you are fully prepared for the future expansion of your uterus.

Core muscles

Your core muscles (which include your abdominals) support your trunk and help maintain good posture; they also link the two halves of your body to provide stability and efficient, safe movement. Ensuring that the core muscles are strong and durable prior to pregnancy, and maintaining their function during pregnancy, is important because they will help to:

- support the back and reduce back pain
- maintain correct pelvic alignment – avoiding poor posture and reducing back and neck pain
- support the increasing weight of your baby
- assist the uterus during labour
- together with a strong pelvic floor, reduce the incidence of stress incontinence.

In addition to the positive health benefits of a strong core, the better the condition of your core before and during pregnancy, the faster you will regain your shape post-partum.

> **Did you know . . .** 90 per cent of pregnant women experience back pain during pregnancy? Maintaining a strong, stable core reduces back pain.

Core strength and stability exercises: trimester 1

The following exercises are designed specifically for trimester 1 and are based on existing advice, but, in general, if you have worked on your core up to conception, you can undertake normal core conditioning throughout trimester 1 (if you are having twins, I recommend starting with trimester 2 exercises). As your baby and uterus are small and well protected inside your abdominal cavity throughout the first trimester, it is unlikely that you could harm your baby with standard core exercises if executed correctly. In contrast, if you have poor core strength and stability, have not worked on your core before getting pregnant, or if you are unsure of any of the exercises, make sure you seek expert advice from an exercise professional before starting out.

Each exercise should be controlled and completed slowly at all times. Because of the low intensity of core strength and stability exercises, you can choose to perform these exercises daily, although two to three times per week should ensure you maintain your core during the first trimester.

If you experience any pain or unusual/uncomfortable feelings, stop the exercise immediately. Keep well hydrated, avoid getting too hot and at all times remember to listen to your body. It is unlikely that you will significantly raise your heart rate during these exercises but it is still worth keeping an eye on it (see 'Use your head' in Chapter 2 to learn about monitoring your heartbeat).

CORE STRENGTH AND STABILITY: TRIMESTER 1

1 Bum lift

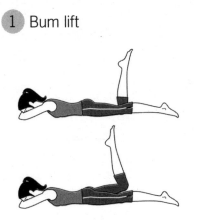

- Lie face down on the floor
- Draw your belly button towards your back and tense your legs and bottom
- Bend your right leg at the knee to 90°
- Raise your right thigh while keeping your hips in contact with the ground
- Hold for 5 seconds
- Return to start position and repeat 10 times
- Repeat for your left leg

2 Side lift

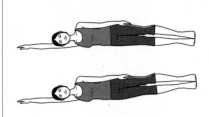

- Lie on your right side with your lower arm extended above your head and your upper arm resting on your side
- Draw your belly button towards your back and tense your legs and bottom
- Straighten your body and, without falling forwards or backwards, lift both legs by about 15cm, keeping your legs straight (if you find two legs too difficult, only lift your upper leg)
- Return to start position and repeat 10 times
- Roll over and repeat on your left side

3 Cushion squeeze

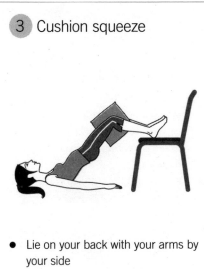

- Lie on your back with your arms by your side
- Place both heels on a chair and with your knees bent at 90° fully extend your hips to form a straight line from your shoulders to hips to knees
- Place a firm cushion between your knees
- Draw your belly button towards your back and tense your legs and bottom
- Squeeze your knees together and hold for 5 seconds
- Repeat 20 times

4 Side lift

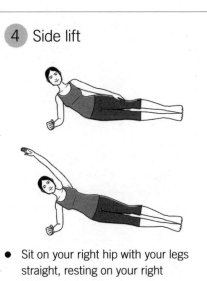

- Sit on your right hip with your legs straight, resting on your right elbow
- Draw your belly button towards your back and tense your legs and bottom
- Without collapsing your arm, lift your hip to the ceiling with your feet on the ground, making a straight line from shoulder to hip to ankle
- Extend your left arm above your head and hold for 10 seconds
- Return to start position and repeat 3 times
- Roll over and repeat on your left hip

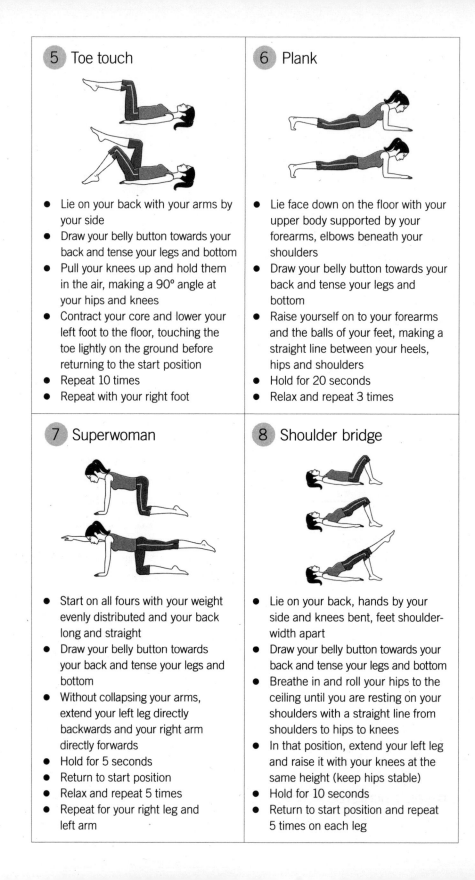

5 Toe touch

- Lie on your back with your arms by your side
- Draw your belly button towards your back and tense your legs and bottom
- Pull your knees up and hold them in the air, making a 90° angle at your hips and knees
- Contract your core and lower your left foot to the floor, touching the toe lightly on the ground before returning to the start position
- Repeat 10 times
- Repeat with your right foot

6 Plank

- Lie face down on the floor with your upper body supported by your forearms, elbows beneath your shoulders
- Draw your belly button towards your back and tense your legs and bottom
- Raise yourself on to your forearms and the balls of your feet, making a straight line between your heels, hips and shoulders
- Hold for 20 seconds
- Relax and repeat 3 times

7 Superwoman

- Start on all fours with your weight evenly distributed and your back long and straight
- Draw your belly button towards your back and tense your legs and bottom
- Without collapsing your arms, extend your left leg directly backwards and your right arm directly forwards
- Hold for 5 seconds
- Return to start position
- Relax and repeat 5 times
- Repeat for your right leg and left arm

8 Shoulder bridge

- Lie on your back, hands by your side and knees bent, feet shoulder-width apart
- Draw your belly button towards your back and tense your legs and bottom
- Breathe in and roll your hips to the ceiling until you are resting on your shoulders with a straight line from shoulders to hips to knees
- In that position, extend your left leg and raise it with your knees at the same height (keep hips stable)
- Hold for 10 seconds
- Return to start position and repeat 5 times on each leg

Your pelvic floor

The pelvic floor muscles contain both fast (power) and slow (endurance) muscle fibres and are found at the base of your abdomen, attached to your pelvis. The pelvic floor is shaped like a sling to support your bowel, uterus and bladder. The action of the pelvic floor muscles controls your vagina, rectum and urethra.

Having a weak pelvic floor makes it harder for you to squeeze the muscles and sphincters at the bottom of your bladder (surrounding the urethra) to prevent wee from escaping. If your pelvic floor is weak, you may accidentally leak a little wee when you cough, sneeze or exercise. This is termed 'stress incontinence', which is particularly common post-partum. With the increasing weight of the uterus pressing on the pelvic floor and the bladder, it is not uncommon to experience leaking during pregnancy. While this may be common and have limited physical health consequences, it can significantly affect your confidence and emotional and psychological health. It is therefore important to maintain the strength of your pelvic floor muscles throughout your pregnancy. In addition to reducing incontinence, exercising your pelvic floor muscles will help you during the delivery of your baby, as you'll be able to better control your pelvis during labour.

Exercising the pelvic floor muscles can be difficult and they are often neglected while we instead engage the abdominals, gluteals (buttocks) and quadriceps (thighs). In order to focus on the pelvic floor muscles, we should think of these muscles as the ones we contract to stop us weeing. Specifically activating the pelvic floor muscles without contracting other muscles is the most efficient way of ensuring you are targeting and improving the strength of the pelvic floor.

Pelvic floor exercises

- Sit or lie comfortably.
- Squeeze the pelvic floor muscles by slowly contracting, holding your maximum contraction for 1 to 2 seconds and then slowly releasing.
- Do not hold your breath or tighten your stomach, buttock or thigh muscles at the same time.
- Once you have mastered the routine of holding the contraction for 1 to 2 seconds, you can move on to the slow-twitch or fast-twitch exercises. By targeting both the slow- and fast-twitch fibres, you will optimize the improvement in pelvic floor strength, endurance and control.

Slow-twitch pelvic floor muscles

- Repeat the exercise above 10 times in a row with around 5 seconds' rest between contractions.
- Once you are able to complete this correctly, start to increase the length of time you hold the contraction. Work up to 10–second holds.
- Remember to make sure you contract and release slowly and under control.
- As you become an advanced exerciser, try releasing the contraction to the halfway point, hold and then fully release slowly.
- You can also increase the number of repetitions but don't overdo it and make sure you rest between sets of contractions.
- You should start to notice the results of your work with greater control and reduced incontinence episodes within a month of starting the exercises.

Fast-twitch pelvic floor muscles

- Contract your pelvic floor muscles and hold your maximum contraction for 1 second and then release.
- Repeat 10 times in a row, with around 5 seconds' rest between contractions or until you feel tired.

Pelvic floor exercises require a great deal of concentration to ensure you are executing them correctly. Do not continue exercising if you start to lose quality, contract other muscles or start holding your breath. Pelvic floor exercises should be part of your daily exercise programme throughout pregnancy and beyond. And do make sure you carry on doing the exercises even when you notice them starting to work. The wonderful thing about pelvic floor exercises is that no one knows you are doing them, so you are free to work out almost anywhere – at the bus stop, waiting at the supermarket checkout or while out for lunch with your friends!

The exercise programme for trimester 1

Being active during pregnancy is crucial for your health and the health of your baby. Exercise will have positive effects on your physical, emotional and social well-being and will ultimately improve your quality of life. Rather than thinking just about discrete periods of the day when you exercise, you should try to be as active as possible throughout the day. Don't sit down for prolonged periods of time and try to make activity part of your daily life. For example, take the stairs rather than the lift and park further away from the entrance to work or the shops. Making these simple changes can dramatically increase your activity levels and improve your health.

That said, exercise in addition to activity is also important, but how much exercise should you be doing? Here are some simple guidelines that reflect the maximum amount of exercise you should aim for – and remember, how much you do during your pregnancy will depend on how much you did before you became pregnant.

EXERCISE IN TRIMESTER 1

Aerobic:	30 minutes at least 5 days per week
Strength:	1 to 2 sessions per week (30 minutes in duration)
Core strength and stability:	2 to 3 sessions per week
Pelvic floor:	daily

Take an extra day for recovery if you are feeling tired and never exercise when you are feeling ill or against your health professional's advice.

Trimester 1 FAQs

Is it safe to swim while I'm pregnant?

Definitely. Swimming will help you maintain your fitness throughout your pregnancy and beyond. It is one of the best exercises you can take, with the water providing a safe and warm environment. The level of the hormone relaxin in your body is yet to lead to significant laxity in your joints, so even breaststroke (which is not recommended during trimester 3; see Chapter 5) is fine to do in the first trimester. Once again, listen to your body and if you experience hip or lower back pain, choose a more suitable stroke.

Is diastasis (splitting of the *linea alba*) painful?

Not usually. Because the *linea alba* is connective tissue, which contains a limited number of pain receptors, and the splitting process occurs over a prolonged period of time, you rarely experience pain. The resultant back pain if you do not maintain your core strength can be much more problematic!

Is stress bad for my baby?

Stress is a part of everyday life. Normally, we are able to cope with daily stresses, which tend to be intermittent and short-lived. In fact, stress can often help to improve performance. In general, if you handle these 'normal' episodes of stress well and they do not become prolonged and debilitating, it is likely that you will cope well with normal levels of stress during your pregnancy. Of course, coping with stress is an entirely individual and personal matter and you should decide for yourself if you feel the stress you are experiencing is overwhelming you and causing you to feel unwell. If you're experiencing symptoms such as anxiety, sleeplessness, negative mood (depression), headaches, loss of appetite or nausea, fatigue/exhaustion, you should think about how you can better manage stressful situations. Also, if you find yourself picking up unhealthy habits from your pre-pregnancy days, for example smoking or drinking alcohol, then it is probably time to make a change.

Remember, it's not just a case of removing the stress, which sometimes is not possible; it is more a question of how to manage or reduce stress during this important time of your life.

There are lots of ways to help reduce stress but adopting a healthy lifestyle is probably the most effective. Exercise in general helps to moderate stress but meditative activities such as yoga (see pages 97 and 136), meditation and mindfulness can be particularly helpful in providing you with the space and time to deal with anxiety.

Eating healthily can also be extremely beneficial, because if you eat well during pregnancy you will provide yourself with the fuel you need to keep you feeling fit and energized now and in the future. It goes without saying that your baby will benefit too! It is likely that you will feel more stressed in your second and third trimesters, so taking control now will help you manage better over the coming months (and years!).

If you have feelings of anxiety or low mood that feel overwhelming, you should always seek help from your healthcare team. This is not something that you should feel embarrassed about, as you are going through a period of immense hormonal and physical change, which can be difficult to cope with.

Does exercise reduce blood flow to my baby?

There appears to be no lasting effect of exercise on the transplacental (across the placenta) transportation of oxygen, carbon dioxide or nutrients. In other words, there is no evidence that moderate-intensity exercise affects the foetus.

Does my baby's heart rate increase when I exercise?

Research has demonstrated that a baby's heart rate can increase by up to 30 beats per minute during or immediately following exercise. Interestingly, the heart rate can also decrease in some instances. The reason for this is not fully understood but these changes in your baby's heart rate during exercise have no negative lasting effect.

PREGNANCY TRIVIA

The powerhouse of life

The mitochondria are the parts of cells that produce the energy for life. It is interesting to note that the mitochondria of the sperm are found in its tail. On entry into the egg, the tail of the sperm is left outside, meaning that while our chromosomes share a contribution from both mother and father (half from each), the mitochondria are entirely maternal. In other words, the mother is wholly responsible for powering life!

Eat your greens

Recent research from Africa (Gambia to be precise) has demonstrated that eating green leafy vegetables during the first trimester has a positive effect on the developing foetus. In general, fruit and vegetables provide important vitamins, minerals and fibre. Green leafy vegetables, which are a rich source of folate (folic acid) and a number of vitamins and minerals, have been shown to support healthy development of the foetus and, together with a variety of fruit and vegetables, improve birth weight.

Hot baby

Your baby's core (body) temperature is about 1°C higher than your own.

Swimming in the blood

Immersion in water results in the redistribution of fluid from outside your cells into your vascular system. In other words, your blood volume increases when you are in water. The increase in blood volume is associated with how deep you go and this is why scuba diving is not recommended during pregnancy – due to the significant increase in blood volume and resultant increase in blood pressure. In contrast, for swimming and aquarobics the smaller increase in blood volume may actually protect your baby from any reduction in blood flow.

4

The Second Trimester:
Months 4 to 6

You and your bump

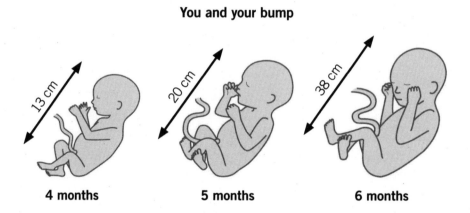

| 4 months | 5 months | 6 months |

The start of trimester 2 will see the foetus growing in length as the spine and neck begin to fully form and straighten. Midway through month 4, your baby starts to look increasingly like a human being, as the ears and eyes move to their recognizable positions. In addition, your baby will start to flex its muscles, moving much more frequently in a coordinated way, although these movements will still be too small for you to feel.

During the second trimester, your baby's brainstem develops to control critical reflexes such as breathing and heart rate, which is now around 140 to 150 beats per minute. By the end of month 4, your baby will have grown to 13cm in length and will weigh around 150g. One of the more unusual developments during this month is the growth of downy hair, called lanugo, over your baby's body. The role of this hairy overcoat is to keep the baby warm and it will gradually disappear as subcutaneous (below-the-skin) fat is laid down over the coming months.

Month 5 witnesses a massive increase in the size of your baby – up to around 450g in weight and to approximately 20cm in length. It is around this time that you will begin to show more prominently and it is likely that you will have a football-sized bump. During month 5, you will also begin to feel your baby's movements for the first time. In addition to practising breathing and swallowing, which began in month 4, your baby is now hiccupping and yawning. To protect your baby from the effects of being suspended in amniotic fluid, a waxy protective layer called *vernix caseosa* is secreted over his or her hairy lanugo overcoat.

The middle of month 5 is marked by your 20-week scan, and now you will notice that the tiny foetus really does begin to look like a baby. By the end of month 5, your baby is starting to develop senses: sight, hearing, taste and touch. And while the baby's eyes are still fused shut, at this point he or she will be able to detect changes in light and will hear the world around them – both inside and outside the womb. They will taste the changes in the amniotic fluid; these changes relate to the food you eat and drink, so it is important to remember to eat and drink healthily!

Month 6 marks the end of trimester 2 and the beginning of another growth spurt as your baby increases its weight to nearly 1kg and its length to 38cm (which is now measured head to toe). By this time not only will you be able to feel the movement of your baby but these movements are also likely to be visible on the surface – which is cute or a bit freaky, depending which way you look at it! This is likely to be the month when you see your own weight begin to increase in relation to the size of your bump.

What symptoms can I expect in the second trimester of pregnancy?

Trimester 2 is often described as the most comfortable, both physically and psychologically, of the three trimesters. Importantly, some of the symptoms that might have been front and centre of your first trimester, i.e. nausea and sickness, and the frequent trips to the toilet, may finally be easing off. In addition, you're likely to feel less fatigued and will have greater energy. That said, you will still experience a host of physical and emotional changes. Again, the individual nature of pregnancy means that you may experience some, none or all of these changes. Indeed, you may have other less common symptoms that are not reported in books, magazines or online. It is important to remember that if you have any concerns at all you should speak with your healthcare professional. The following are common changes that you may experience.

PHYSICAL AND EMOTIONAL CHANGES: TRIMESTER 2			
	Month 4	**Month 5**	**Month 6**
PHYSICAL			
Fatigue (often less than trimester 1)	✓		
Increased energy levels (compared with trimester 1)		✓	✓
Decreased nausea and vomiting	✓	✓	✓
Bloating, flatulence, indigestion, heartburn, reflux	✓	✓	✓
Increasing frequency of urination	✓	✓	✓
Constipation	✓	✓	✓

	Month 4	Month 5	Month 6
Continued enlargement of breasts, often with reduced tenderness	✓	✓	✓
Vaginal discharge	✓ small amounts	✓	✓
Development of varicose veins and haemorrhoids	✓	✓	✓
Increased heart rate		✓	✓
Minor foot and ankle swelling	✓	✓	✓
Leg cramps (mainly in calves)		✓	✓
Occasional headaches	✓	✓	✓
Occasional dizziness and light-headedness	✓	✓	✓
Increased appetite	✓	✓	✓
Bunged-up nose and ears (possible occasional nosebleed) due to increased hormone levels causing inflammation of your nasal passages	✓	✓	✓
Gum sensitivity (possible bleeding during brushing) due to build-up of plaque associated with hormonal changes (sometimes called 'pregnancy gingivitis')	✓	✓	✓
Growth of your bump	✓	✓	✓
Pain in abdomen associated with stretching due to increased size of the uterus		✓	✓

	Month 4	Month 5	Month 6
Skin pigmentation changes on stomach and face (darkening of skin termed 'chloasma' is due to hormones increasing melanin production) and stretch marks		✓	✓
Back ache			✓
Protruding belly button		✓	✓
Foetal movement		✓	✓ observable from outside
EMOTIONAL			
Mood swings, irritability, irrationality, unexpected crying (heightened premenstrual syndrome) associated with hormone changes	✓	✓	✓ fewer mood swings
Forgetfulness		✓	✓

Exercise and the second trimester

Exercise should remain a central part of your life throughout trimester 2 of your pregnancy. The same positive health benefits exercise provided you with in trimester 1 remain; however, during trimester 2, as your baby begins to grow more rapidly, the importance of maintaining your aerobic conditioning, strength (including your core and pelvic floor) and mobility increases. If you maintained your exercise programme throughout trimester 1, you will only need to make minor modifications in trimester 2.

The biggest change affecting your exercise routine in trimester 2 is the ever-increasing size of your bump and breasts, which results in elevated stress on your pelvic floor and abdominal muscles, and an altered centre of gravity, leading to postural changes. These changes, together with the increased workload of carrying your baby, mean you will have to change the position of some exercises (for example, avoid lying on your back), modify or cut out others (such as sit-ups) and reduce the speed at which you work and the weights that you lift in order to maintain moderate intensity. It is also advisable to avoid risky exercises, in particular those that increase the potential for falling and impact. And, as always, listen to your body and stop immediately if you have any concerns or discomfort and speak with your healthcare team.

Aerobic exercise

With the increasing weight of your uterus placing pressure on your pelvic floor and your back, you might want to think about reducing, and eventually stopping, intense bouncing or jumping-type exercises such as skipping by the end of trimester 2. Even running might be a bit too much for some as trimester 2 progresses, so think carefully and listen to your body before continuing to run. Of course, if you are very well conditioned and have a history of running, you can continue through trimester 2 and into trimester 3, although your intensity (speed) should be reduced in line with the general guidelines (see Chapter 2).

In general, the types of exercises that you can do in trimester 2 are the same as trimester 1. The only exception may be rowing, which is entirely safe (as long as you have good technique) but you may find that your bump starts to get in the way!

The duration of exercise required to maintain health and performance remains at around 30 minutes; however, you may, on occasion, feel 30 minutes is too long. But don't worry – rather than giving it a miss, simply divide the session into smaller, more manageable chunks.

Research has shown that three 10-minute bouts of aerobic exercise spread across the day are as effective as a single 30-minute session.

Remember to always keep a check on the intensity of your exercise. The advice to keep your RPE at or below 7 (or 75 per cent of your maximum heart rate) remains appropriate throughout your pregnancy (see Chapter 2). The difference is what you can do before you reach an RPE of 7. As your body changes, you are likely to find that moderate-intensity exercise is reached at slower speeds in trimester 2 than it was in trimester 1, so make sure you modify your workout to accommodate these changes.

Listen to your body and change your exercise routine accordingly. Every day will feel different, so don't worry or get anxious about altering your plan to suit how you feel (physically and psychologically); just remember, any exercise is good for mind, body and soul. You don't even have to leave the house to benefit from some aerobic exercise. On the following pages is a simple aerobic exercise programme you can do wherever you are – no fancy equipment or gym membership required!

AEROBIC EXERCISES: TRIMESTER 2

You can complete these exercises without weights. If you choose to use dumbbells, you should select a weight with which you can complete all the repetitions of each exercise. Use the same weight throughout and consider increasing the weight of your dumbbells when you can easily complete all exercises.

Always complete the exercises slowly and under control. Move through the exercises at your own pace but without resting between exercises. Remember to keep your RPE at 7 or below, avoid overheating and have fluid with you to drink when required.

1 Squat

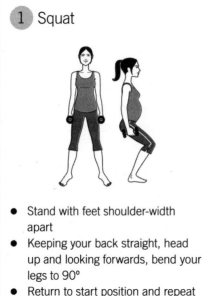

- Stand with feet shoulder-width apart
- Keeping your back straight, head up and looking forwards, bend your legs to 90°
- Return to start position and repeat 20 times

2 Push-ups

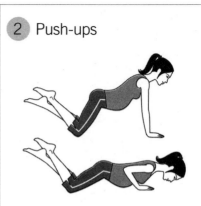

- Start on all fours with your legs bent, knees together, ankles crossed and arms outstretched with hands shoulder-width apart
- Form a straight line from your head to your knees
- Draw your belly button towards your back and tense your legs and bottom
- Lower your body to the floor
- When your arms are at 90°, pause and straighten your arms
- Repeat 20 times

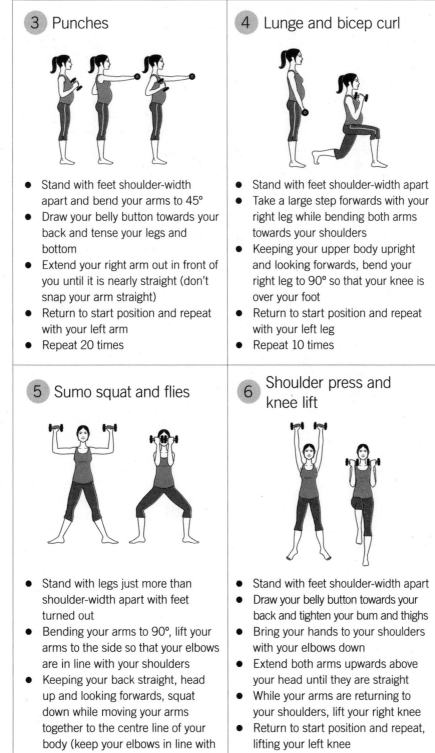

3 Punches

- Stand with feet shoulder-width apart and bend your arms to 45°
- Draw your belly button towards your back and tense your legs and bottom
- Extend your right arm out in front of you until it is nearly straight (don't snap your arm straight)
- Return to start position and repeat with your left arm
- Repeat 20 times

4 Lunge and bicep curl

- Stand with feet shoulder-width apart
- Take a large step forwards with your right leg while bending both arms towards your shoulders
- Keeping your upper body upright and looking forwards, bend your right leg to 90° so that your knee is over your foot
- Return to start position and repeat with your left leg
- Repeat 10 times

5 Sumo squat and flies

- Stand with legs just more than shoulder-width apart with feet turned out
- Bending your arms to 90°, lift your arms to the side so that your elbows are in line with your shoulders
- Keeping your back straight, head up and looking forwards, squat down while moving your arms together to the centre line of your body (keep your elbows in line with your shoulders)
- Return to start position and repeat 20 times

6 Shoulder press and knee lift

- Stand with feet shoulder-width apart
- Draw your belly button towards your back and tighten your bum and thighs
- Bring your hands to your shoulders with your elbows down
- Extend both arms upwards above your head until they are straight
- While your arms are returning to your shoulders, lift your right knee
- Return to start position and repeat, lifting your left knee
- Repeat 20 times

7 Side bend

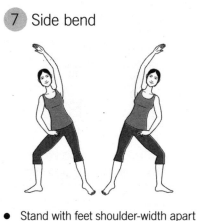

- Stand with feet shoulder-width apart
- Draw your belly button towards your back and tense your legs and bottom
- Extend your left arm above your head and towards the right, bending at the hip (do not bend forwards or backwards)
- Return to start position and repeat with your right arm
- Repeat 20 times

8 Squat and push press

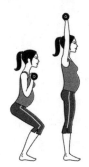

- Stand upright with feet shoulder-width apart with soft knees
- Bring your hands to your shoulders with your elbows down
- Keeping your back straight, head up and looking forwards, bend the legs to 90°
- As you stand, extend both arms upwards above your head until they are straight
- Return to start position and repeat 20 times

9 Twists

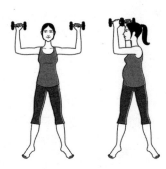

- Stand with feet shoulder-width apart
- Draw your belly button towards your back and tense your legs and bottom
- Bend your arms to 90° and lift your arms to the side until your elbows are level with your shoulders
- Keeping your back straight and head up, rotate around to your right
- Return to start position and repeat, rotating around to your left
- Repeat 20 times

Take a dip

Water workouts become increasingly enjoyable as your bump grows. In water, you and your bump feel considerably lighter than on land, which can make swimming, aquarobics, deep-water walking or even running an escape from the work of carrying your extra cargo. Your near weightlessness in water offloads the pressure on your joints, including your back, while being a fabulous way to focus on your aerobic fitness.

In addition, the added resistance offered by the water will help develop your strength and strength endurance in a safe and supported environment. As water is 25 times more conductive than air (water takes away heat much faster) you are also much less likely to overheat.

> **Top Tip: Don't get hot under the collar!** Avoid overheating during exercise. Wear layers so that you can peel them off as you begin to warm up and make sure you always have adequate fluid with you.

Strength exercise

Using weights or bands to increase resistance remains an important part of your exercise programme throughout trimester 2. Strong muscles will support your increasingly lax joints and reduce the associated pain. In addition, maintaining strength will help you cope with your rapidly growing baby and make normal daily activities much easier and safer!

You will only need to make minor modifications to your trimester 1 strength programme in trimester 2, the most important of which is a reduction in the weight you lift. As always, the changes you need to make will depend on your experience and your current level of conditioning. If you were using machine or free weights prior to becoming pregnant and during trimester 1, you can continue these exercises throughout trimester 2 by simply reducing the weight you lift (it is advisable to change from barbells to dumbbells). If strength exercise is not your forte, then you can use bands to create resistance (see the following pages for examples of exercises using bands).

The change in your centre of gravity associated with the increased weight and size of your bump and breasts can make you a little more unstable during trimester 2. For that reason, you should take care to ensure good technique and posture, and maintain control throughout each exercise.

Avoiding or modifying the following exercises is advisable in trimester 2:

- exercises that directly work your abdominals, i.e. sit-ups
- lying on your back (reduce duration and/or modify exercises)
- lying on your tummy
- exercises that require rapid twisting or rapid changes in direction
- high-impact exercises
- anaerobic exercise (keep it at an RPE of 7 or below)
- contact sports
- excessive range of motion, including deep squats (normal squats to 90° are OK)
- risky exercises – those which increase the chances of falling or impact, i.e. skiing, horse riding or combat sports.

7 is the magic number! Remember to always maintain an RPE of 7 or below during exercise. Alter your speed and the weights you are lifting to keep you in the zone at all times.

1 Squat

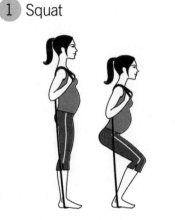

- Place the middle of the band under your feet, hold a handle firmly in each hand and bring each length up over your shoulders
- Draw your belly button towards your back and tense your legs and bottom
- Stand with feet shoulder-width apart and arms bent, with hands touching your shoulders, palms facing forwards and elbows touching your sides
- Keeping your back straight and looking forwards, bend the legs to 90°
- Return to start position and repeat 20 times

2 Biceps curl

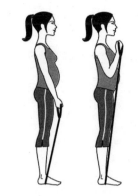

- Place the middle of the band under your feet and hold a handle firmly in each hand
- Draw your belly button towards your back and tense your legs and bottom
- Stand with feet shoulder-width apart and hands on the front of your thighs with palms facing forwards
- Bend the arms to bring the hands to the chest, keeping your elbows against your side
- Return to start position and repeat 20 times

3 Leg extension

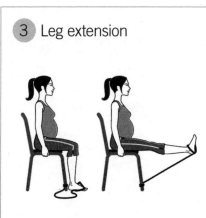

- Place the band behind the front legs of a chair, looping the band around its legs
- Sitting upright looking forwards, hold the sides of the chair firmly
- Place a foot through each handle
- Extend both legs straight in front of you, forming a straight line from your hip to knee to ankle
- Return to start position and repeat 20 times

4 Shoulder press

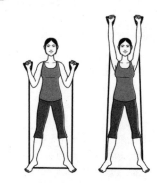

- Place the middle of the band under your feet and hold a handle firmly in each hand
- Stand with feet shoulder-width apart and arms bent, hands at shoulder height with elbows down
- Extend both arms upwards above your head until they are straight
- Return to start position and repeat 20 times

5 Leg curl

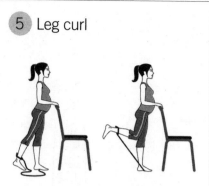

- Place your right foot through the handle and stand on the band with your left foot, adjusting the tension to create a medium resistance
- Stand upright looking forwards with feet shoulder-width apart
- Draw your belly button towards your back and tense your legs and bottom
- Hold a chair or the wall to stabilize the body
- Lift your right lower leg behind you as high as possible, aiming to touch the heel of your foot on your bum
- Return to start position and repeat 20 times
- Repeat for your left leg

6 Clam

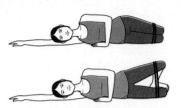

- Wrap the band securely around your knees, leaving a small length of band between the knees requiring a hard extension of the band to lift the knee
- Lie on your right side with your lower arm extended above your head and your upper arm in front of you supporting your body
- Keep the legs together, bent at 90°, making a straight line from your shoulders to hips to knees
- Keeping the feet together, lift your left knee as high as possible
- Return to start position
- Repeat 20 times
- Turn over and repeat with your right leg on top

7 Kick

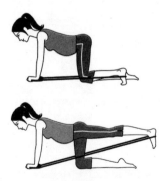

- Start on all fours with your weight evenly distributed
- Hold the handles of the band firmly and place the middle of the band on the sole of the left foot
- Extend your left leg straight behind you and lift the straight leg upwards as high as possible without turning out the hip
- Return to start position and repeat 20 times
- Repeat for your right leg

Core strength and stability

Your baby and your uterus are growing fast during trimester 2 and as your bump grows it will progressively increase the stress it places on your core muscles. This added stress can lead to a dull aching feeling around your trunk and can reduce the strength of your core. At the same time, the extra weight you are carrying out front will begin to place an ever-increasing strain on your back as your posture changes. It is important that you continue to maintain the strength of your core muscles during trimester 2 to help your posture and reduce the all-too-common back-pain blues!

Exercises that involve lying on your back become more problematic from trimester 2 onwards. While there is no significant effect on your baby, the weight of your uterus pressing on your back and a variety of organs and blood vessels makes lying on your back uncomfortable. (Of course, lying on your front is even more uncomfortable!) In addition, if you are suffering from dizziness and light-headedness, lying on your back to exercise can make matters worse. Although it is rare, you may suffer from supine hypotensive syndrome, where your blood pressure falls dramatically when you lie on your back (compressing blood vessels and reducing blood flow), leading to dizziness, light-headedness and occasional syncope (fainting). If you suffer from this syndrome, you should avoid exercising on your back. If you have no such problems, you can continue exercising on your back but aim for short periods of time and think about using cushions/pillows to prop you up (avoid sitting up using your abs; use your arms to change position or roll on to your side before getting up).

Special considerations during trimester 2

- Avoid 'doming' your abdominals. Make sure you contract your abdominals throughout exercise; do not allow them to be stretched outwards.

- Be careful when getting down to and up from the floor or when changing positions. Make sure you contract your abdominals and use your arms to assist you.

- Remember, you should ensure that each exercise is controlled and completed slowly at all times.

- Daily core strength and stability exercise is fine but 2 to 3 times per week should ensure you maintain your core strength and stability.

- Work at your own pace, don't rush, and listen to your body.

Top Tip: And breathe! Breathing is an important part of strength, and core strength and stability exercise. Make sure you concentrate on your breathing by slowly exhaling during contractions. Do not hold your breath; while this is unlikely to be a problem for your baby, it may lead to light-headedness and dizziness for you.

Mind the gap!

As we learned in the previous chapter, your abs will come under increasing pressure as your bump grows. Importantly, during the second trimester your *linea alba* (the band of connective tissue running down the middle of your abs) will start to be stretched as the connective tissue begins to soften and your bump grows. It is very common for the *linea alba* to begin to split at this time in a process called diastasis. This is particularly true, and more common, if you're not a first-timer. There is nothing to be concerned about, as this almost entirely painless process is a natural part of pregnancy. Diastasis usually starts at the belly button and then moves either up or down the abdominals. You can sometimes feel the gap when you are lying down by placing your fingers on your tummy just below or above your belly button.

While there is very little you can do to avoid diastasis, there are exercises that may place undue pressure on the abdominals and accelerate the process. It is best to avoid exercises that specifically focus on the abdominals during trimester 2, including sit-ups, crunches and leg raises. By improving all of your core muscles you can better support the increasing weight of your bump and reduce the stress on your abs.

Top Tip: Pelvic floor, pelvic floor, pelvic floor! If you do nothing else, make sure you continue with your pelvic floor exercises. As the weight of your uterus increases, the stress on your pelvic floor intensifies, leading to an increasing incontinence problem. And remember, your pelvic floor is not just for now; you'll be thankful for a strong pelvic floor during and after delivery!

CORE STRENGTH AND STABILITY: TRIMESTER 2

1 Cushion squeeze

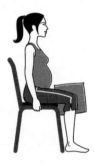

- In a seated position, place a firm cushion between your knees
- Squeeze your knees together and hold for 5 seconds
- Repeat 10 times

2 Side lift

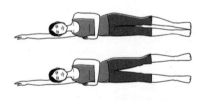

- Lie on your right side with your lower arm extended above your head and your upper arm in front of you supporting your body
- Draw your belly button towards your back and tense your legs and bottom
- Straighten your body and, without falling forwards or backwards, lift your left leg by about 15cm, keeping your leg straight
- Return to start position and repeat 10 times
- Roll over and repeat for your right leg

3 Bum lift

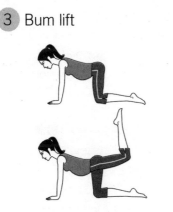

- Start on all fours with your weight evenly distributed
- Draw your belly button towards your back and tense your legs and bottom
- Without collapsing your arms, lift your left leg directly upwards – imagine your toes are being pulled by a string straight up to the ceiling
- Hold for 5 seconds
- Return to start position and repeat 10 times
- Repeat for your right leg

4 Shoulder bridge

- Lie on your back, hands by your side and knees bent, feet shoulder-width apart
- Draw your belly button towards your back and tense your legs and bottom
- Breathe in and roll your hips to the ceiling until you are resting on your shoulders with a straight line from shoulders to hips to knees
- Hold for 10 seconds
- Return to start position and repeat 10 times

5 Side lift

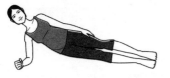

- Sit on your right hip, resting on your right elbow with your legs straight
- Draw your belly button towards your back and tense your legs and bottom
- Without collapsing your arm, lift your hips to make a straight line from shoulder to hip to ankle
- Hold for 20 seconds
- Return to start position and repeat 10 times
- Roll over and repeat for your left hip

6 Plank

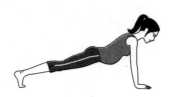

- Start on all fours with your weight evenly distributed
- Draw your belly button towards your back and tense your legs and bottom
- Move into a press-up position, making a straight line between your heels, hips and shoulders
- Hold for 20 seconds
- Relax and repeat 5 times

7 Toe touch

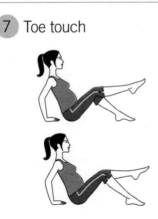

- Sit on the floor with your hands behind you to support your upper body
- Draw your belly button towards your back and tense your legs and bottom
- Bend your legs to 90°
- Lift your right knee towards your chest before returning to start position
- Repeat 10 times
- Repeat for your left knee

8 Cat

- Start on all fours with your weight evenly distributed
- Draw your belly button towards your back and tense your legs and bottom
- Allowing your head to drop, slowly arch your back upwards and hold momentarily
- Return to start position and repeat 10 times

9 Clam

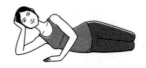

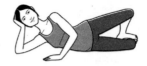

- Lie on your right side with your spine aligned with the edge of your mat, your lower arm bent at the elbow to support your head and your upper arm in front of you supporting your body
- Stack your legs one on top of the other and bend your knees to 90°
- Keeping your feet together, lift your left knee as high as possible
- Return to start position and repeat 10 times
- Roll over and repeat for your right knee
  (You could use your elasticated band wrapped around your knees to increase the resistance)

And relax . . . Yoga is a fabulous form of exercise during pregnancy. Not only is it low intensity and low impact, yoga can also provide some much-needed time, space and quiet for a little mindfulness. Remember, however, the hormone relaxin has made you much more supple, so avoid over-stretching beyond your normal (pre-pregnancy) range of motion. Also, take care with yoga in hot environments (e.g. Bikram yoga) to avoid overheating. As always, drink plenty of water as you exercise.

Sexercise!

Sex is generally safe throughout pregnancy, and while your libido can change dramatically from trimester to trimester (and from day to day!) due to the dramatic fluctuations in hormones, physical changes in your body and disturbances in mood, sex can be a fun and enjoyable form of exercise.

Sadly, the myth that one expends a good deal of energy during sex simply isn't true. While there are obvious positional changes that have higher or lower energy expenditures, in general you only burn around 100 calories during sex, although much depends on how long you last. While your chosen position may govern your energy expenditure, it is much more likely to be comfort that dictates your preferred position, and this will change throughout pregnancy. Although not always the case, it is likely that during trimester 2 your interest in sex will be at its peak, so make the most of this enjoyable part of your exercise programme!

Top Tip: Just a little nudge. Improving your pelvic floor muscles will increase your sensitivity during sex – another good reason to keep up your pelvic floor exercises!

A bumpy night's sleep!

Sleep is of critical importance in maintaining physical, psychological and emotional health; it is a vital period of the day for recovery and growth, so optimizing your sleep quality is crucial for you and your baby. It's not just about how much time you spend in bed; it's about the quality of your sleep. As your baby grows, sleep can become increasingly problematic. In addition to the rise in your body temperature, increased frequency of urination and issues with finding a comfortable position as your bump gets ever larger mean your sleep quality is diminishing by the day. But all is not lost! Adopting good sleep practices can significantly improve the quality of your sleep and, of course, exercise can have a really positive effect too. Here are some tips to help.

- Make sure your bedroom is dark (blackout curtains can really help).
- Keep your bedroom cool.
- Reduce noise as much as possible (earplugs are sometimes a good option).
- Remove all electronic devices from the bedroom (no mobile phones, televisions or tablets).
- Have a warm bath or shower to relax, and brush your teeth before bed.
- Chill out and give yourself an hour to unwind before getting into bed.
- Avoid eating a large meal before bed.
- Avoid coffee (or any caffeinated drinks) for at least a couple of hours before bed.
- Avoid drinking too much close to bedtime (this will help reduce the need to pee!).

Goodnight. People who exercise are much more likely to get to sleep quicker, and sleep deeper and undisturbed; they are also more likely to wake up feeling refreshed. Relaxing exercise close to bedtime, e.g. yoga or a gentle flexibility exercise, can help you to get to sleep quicker.

The exercise programme for trimester 2

Exercise remains as important during trimester 2 as it was in trimester 1. In fact, for many reasons exercise is even more important in trimester 2 and beyond, as the changes in your body begin to accelerate. The increasing size of your bump and breasts, combined with the increased laxity of your joints, makes back and joint pain much more likely. The rising weight of your uterus increases the stress placed on your pelvic floor, and your overall increase in weight together with an altered posture make the activities of daily living a little bit more like hard work. But now is not the time to take it easy on the exercise front; making sure you maintain your core strength and stability, your pelvic floor, your strength and aerobic capacity is key to optimizing your quality of life during trimester 2.

Obviously, during trimester 2 you should begin to adapt your exercise programme to suit your changing needs. With the rapid growth of your baby, some exercises will begin to become less comfortable (or advisable) but rather than simply stopping altogether, think about modifying your routine to accommodate your ever-increasing bump or try something different. While the general advice for intensity of an RPE of 7 or less remains, you will need to reduce your speed and the weights you are lifting to remain in the moderate-intensity zone. If the longer sessions are too much for you, which may be the case during the later stages of trimester 2, don't worry; simply divide your exercise into more manageable chunks – you will still gain the same benefits.

So don't relax for too long on the sofa, stay active and you will maximize all the physical, psychological, emotional and social benefits exercise has to offer.

EXERCISE IN TRIMESTER 2

Aerobic:	30 minutes at least 5 days per week (split into 10-minute bouts spread across the day if you can't manage it in one go)
Strength:	1 to 2 sessions per week (30 minutes in duration or you could try shorter sessions more frequently, i.e. multiple 10-minute sessions spread across the week)
Core strength and stability:	2 to 3 sessions per week
Pelvic floor:	daily

Trimester 2 FAQs

Can I return to exercise if morning sickness and fatigue stopped me in trimester 1?

Definitely. There is nothing to stop you starting exercise at any stage during your pregnancy. The most important issue to consider when starting, or restarting, exercise during pregnancy is to make sure you modify the exercises to take into account your current physical condition. A good rule of thumb is to select exercises from the following trimester (i.e. if you are in trimester 1, start with trimester 2 exercises; if you are in trimester 2, start with trimester 3 exercises). As always, listen to your body and adjust the exercises to suit your own needs.

Why has my posture changed and what can I do about it?

Your centre of gravity is changing! The increasing weight of your bump is all out front, which leads to an exaggerated curving of your lower back (lumbar spine). Add to this the rounding of your upper back (thoracic spine) due to the increased weight of your breasts, and you have the perfect recipe for posture change. Here are some tips to help.

- Draw your shoulder blades back and down (imagine you are trying to put them in your back pockets).
- Stand tall through your spine.
- Draw your chin in and down, and line up your neck with your back.
- Lightly contract your abs.
- Tilt your pelvis towards your belly button (the pelvic tilt).
- Wear a supportive and fitted bra, the size of which will change throughout pregnancy as your breasts change.

Why does my back hurt and what can I do about it?

You have now been releasing the hormone relaxin for over three months, which has resulted in an increasing laxity (softening and stretching) of your tendons and ligaments. This can lead to unstable joints, which together with the increasing weight of your bump and breasts leads to back pain. It is really important that you work on improving your core strength and the strength of your legs, bum and upper back to help stabilize your spine. By combining these measures with improved posture, you can reduce back and neck pain, and reduce the occurrence of headaches. In addition, making sure you are comfortable and well supported when you sleep will help reduce the pressure on your back. Using pillows in a variety of positions (behind your back, between your legs and/or under your bump) can help support you during sleep. Making sure you have the right pillow to support your head and neck will also reduce neck pain and improve sleep quality.

What can I do about constipation during pregnancy?

Exercise combined with a healthy diet rich in fibre can be the only laxative you need during pregnancy. You don't have to work up a sweat to make sure you're regular; even as little as a 10-minute walk will help keep everything moving. In addition to eating foods that are high in fibre, i.e. fresh vegetables and fruit, making sure you are well hydrated will ensure you are creating the right environment in your bowels to help move things along. Don't be afraid of a little coffee to speed things up if you're struggling. Importantly, try to avoid straining when you are on the toilet; haemorrhoids are an issue for many pregnant women and they can be made worse by excessive pushing when constipated.

What is *hyperemesis gravidarum* and will it improve to allow me to start exercising?

Nausea and vomiting is very common during pregnancy; however, *hyperemesis gravidarum* (HG) is at the extreme end of pregnancy sickness, leading to continuous and debilitating nausea and vomiting. While HG is uncommon (affecting about 1 in 200 pregnancies), in some cases it may require hospital treatment. In general, HG begins to subside in month 4; however, it can persist throughout pregnancy. It is important to note that HG is unlikely to affect your baby as long as you follow the advice of your healthcare team. Once your symptoms have improved, you can return to exercise but remember you will have lost some conditioning, so begin easy and build gradually.

What does PGP/SPD stand for and what are the best exercises to deal with it?

Pelvic Girdle Pain (PGP) and Symphysis Pubis Dysfunction (SPD) are terms that describe the same problem (PGP is more commonly used now, as pain is not solely associated with the pubic symphysis – the area at the front of the pelvis). While the problem does not affect your baby, it can cause you misery and significantly reduce your activity levels. Exercises that improve the strength of your pelvic floor and your core strength and stability can reduce the pain and improve function. Water-based exercise is particularly valuable, as the reduced load-bearing and warmth help reduce pain and improve movement. Manual therapy from an experienced practitioner (e.g. a physiotherapist) can help. Being as active as possible, within the limits of pain, is wholly positive in the management of PGP/SPD.

PREGNANCY TRIVIA

You're under arrest!

Your baby is identifiably one of a kind by the beginning of month 5, when he or she develops fingerprints unique to them.

Am I really a boy or a girl?

By the time you have your 20-week scan, your baby's sex organs have already developed. If it's a girl, her uterus has fully formed and her ovaries will already be full of millions of primitive eggs. If it's a boy, he's a bit behind the girls, of course! His testicles have formed and are making their way down to the scrotum, which is still under construction. One thing is for sure, you can spot the difference at 20 weeks – most of the time!

Living at altitude

Your foetus has a 50 per cent higher haemoglobin (the oxygen-carrying part of the red blood cell) content in its blood, with a different formula to us, which means it has a superior ability to transport and supply oxygen. This is important, as the foetus copes with naturally lower oxygen levels in the uterus, which is equivalent to living at altitude!

Pumping iron

It is possible that excessive fatigue during pregnancy can be caused by iron deficiency anaemia. This is particularly true if you have been pregnant in quick succession or you have suffered badly with vomiting or have eaten very little due to morning sickness. While your baby is unlikely to be affected (iron-deficient babies are very uncommon), you may benefit from iron supplementation. Importantly, speak with your healthcare team before starting supplements.

P.S Don't forget your iron-rich foods, such as green leafy vegetables and red meats.

Sugar rush

Gestational diabetes (GD) usually begins around the end of trimester 2 and is associated with an insufficient production of insulin or an insensitivity to insulin that leads to poor control of blood sugar. GD occurs in around 1 in 20 pregnancies and is more common in obese mothers. GD (and diabetes in general) is not harmful to your baby as long as it is well controlled. Exercise and diet are central to reducing the risk of the development of GD and also act as an important treatment for mothers with GD.

Obese women who exercise during pregnancy can reduce their risk of developing GD by 50 per cent!

Bless you

The increased physical and psychological demands of pregnancy can leave you susceptible to coughs and colds. The last thing you need is something else to make you feel under the weather, so make sure you follow these simple steps

- wash your hands regularly
- avoid hand contact with your eyes, nose and mouth
- stay away from infected people; keep well hydrated and eat healthily
- get lots of quality sleep.

It's worth noting that people who exercise regularly have a lower incidence of infection!

5

The Third Trimester: Months 7 to 9

You and your bump

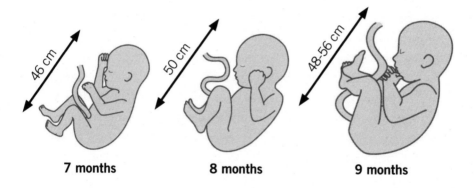

46 cm

50 cm

48-56 cm

7 months　　　　**8 months**　　　　**9 months**

Trimester 3 sees the biggest expansion of your bump as your baby triples or even quadruples in weight from 1kg at the end of trimester 2 to around 4kg at birth (that's as much as 0.25kg per week!). The rapid expansion of your bump is marked by increased aches and pains as your body adapts to the ever-increasing weight of your uterus. In particular, your bump, as well as intensifying the pressure on your pelvic floor, continues to extend out front, further changing your centre of gravity and placing additional stress on your back and hips, which often leads to changes in your gait and that characteristic pregnancy waddle!

As for your baby, development is moving on at a rapid pace, preparing the new arrival for life outside of the womb. By the end of month 7, your baby's lungs will be almost fully developed and his or her brain will be growing rapidly, creating those characteristic folds. At this point, your baby will also be taking control of a variety of functions that, up until recently, it has relied upon you to manage, for example regulating his or her own temperature. Your baby now starts to dream as it sleeps, and with eyelids that can now blink he or she will experience REM (rapid eye movement) sleep – something that you may be struggling with at night! As your baby moves closer to its birth length, much of the increase in weight comes from the laying down of fat that will help keep him or her warm in the outside world. As a result, your baby begins to shed the lanugo overcoat.

Month 8 and the excitement, trepidation and sometimes a little fear may begin to build as you get closer to your due date. This emotional rollercoaster, combined with the ever-increasing physical symptoms as your bump continues to expand, is likely to result in a perpetual feeling of discomfort, day and night. Staying in good physical condition and optimizing your rest and sleep quality will significantly reduce the stress of these later stages of pregnancy.

By the end of month 8, your baby will have reached its birth length and increased in weight to around 2.5kg (remember, every baby is an individual and therefore length and weight will vary). With an increase in size comes diminishing space and you are likely to really feel, and see, your baby's movements. You may also start to feel kicks into your diaphragm and ribs as your baby assumes a head-down position in preparation for the final push.

Month 9, and the final countdown begins. Your baby's weight continues to increase, along with the control of a host of functions that will be valuable in life outside the womb. In fact, almost all of your baby's organs are all systems go (with the exception of the digestive system, which won't switch on until its first feed post-delivery). While you continue to practise your exercises throughout trimester 3, your baby is practising for life outside by moving, sucking, breathing (amniotic fluid at this stage) and blinking. As one of the biggest physical efforts of your life approaches, you'll be glad that you continued your exercise programme throughout your pregnancy and are in great shape for the big day.

What changes can I expect in the third trimester of pregnancy?

The dramatic increase in the weight of your baby (and uterus) during trimester 3 will lead to an increased amount of physical changes compared with trimester 2. The size of your uterus means that you will be feeling aches and pains across your torso from your pelvic floor to your back, and from your stretched abdominals to your lungs with the increased work of breathing. Your emotions will also be heightened as you approach the big day. As with trimesters 1 and 2, the individual nature of pregnancy means that you may experience some, none or all of these changes. Indeed, you may have other less common symptoms that are not reported in books, magazines or online. It is important to remember that if you have any concerns at all, speak with your healthcare professional. Overleaf are common symptoms that you may experience.

PHYSICAL AND EMOTIONAL CHANGES: TRIMESTER 3

	Month 7	Month 8	Month 9
PHYSICAL			
Fatigue	✓	✓	✓
Bloating, flatulence, indigestion, heartburn, reflux	✓	✓	✓
Increased frequency of urination	✓	✓	✓
Constipation	✓	✓	✓
Continued enlargement of breasts	✓	✓	✓
Colostrum leaking from nipples	✓	✓	✓
Vaginal discharge (increased from trimester 2)	✓	✓	✓ heavier with possible red/brown staining
Development of varicose veins and haemorrhoids	✓	✓	✓
Shortness of breath due to your uterus pressing up on your diaphragm (below your lungs)	✓	✓	✓ may improve as baby drops into pelvis
Foot and ankle swelling	✓	✓	✓
Leg cramps (mainly in calves)	✓	✓	✓
Occasional headaches, dizziness and light-headedness	✓	✓	✓
Bunged-up nose and ears (possible occasional nosebleed) due to increased hormones causing inflammation of your nasal passages	✓	✓	✓

	Month 7	Month 8	Month 9
Gum sensitivity (possible bleeding during brushing) due to build-up of plaque associated with hormonal changes (sometimes called 'pregnancy gingivitis')	✓	✓	✓
Growth of your bump	✓	✓	✓
Pain in abdomen associated with stretching due to increased size of the uterus	✓	✓	✓
Stretch marks	✓	✓	✓
Back ache, pelvic discomfort/pain	✓	✓	✓
Protruding belly button	✓	✓	
Foetal movement (stronger and more frequent)	✓ observable from outside	✓ observable from outside	✓ squirming rather than kicking
Braxton Hicks (practice) contractions		✓	✓ more intense, possibly painful
Poor sleep quality	✓	✓	✓
EMOTIONAL			
Mood swings, irritability, irrationality, unexpected crying (heightened premenstrual syndrome) associated with hormone changes	✓	✓	✓
Excitement, anxiety, fear	✓	✓	✓
Forgetfulness	✓	✓	✓

Exercise and the third trimester

It should be business as usual when it comes to exercise in trimester 3. In fact, the benefits of exercise are probably greater in this trimester than in the previous two. As the growth of your baby (and uterus) accelerates in the final stages of pregnancy, it is more important than ever to be as strong and as flexible as possible. Think about trimester 3 as 'the final stretch'. And stretch it is, as your ever-expanding uterus places increasing pressure on your pelvic floor, your abdominal and core muscles, and your back and pelvis. In addition to the increased stretch, the increased weight of your bump will make everyday tasks that much more difficult and tiring, and sleep less likely. But never fear, exercise is the magic pill that can address all of the physical and some of the emotional issues you will face in this final trimester.

As mentioned, maintaining your strength, aerobic endurance, core strength and stability, and flexibility will help you cope better with daily life, help you sleep better and give you something to focus on other than the birth. You will have to make some changes to your exercise programme, including reducing the speed of your activity and the weights you lift, to ensure you stay at or below an RPE of 7, or 75 per cent of maximum heart rate (see Chapter 2). It may also be time to offload and move to non-weight-bearing exercise, for example aquarobics, swimming, cross-trainer or cycling, to reduce the pressure on your pelvis. However, as with trimesters 1 and 2, how you change your programme will depend on your fitness levels coming into trimester 3. And don't forget the omnipresent pelvic floor exercises!

Because of your rapidly changing centre of gravity (due to the forward growth of your bump), balance and coordination may become more of an issue. Accordingly, avoiding or modifying exercises that require these skills is advisable, particularly if loss of balance could lead to a fall. Risky exercises, those which are likely to increase the potential for falling and impact, are much less advisable in trimester 3. And, as always, listen to your body and stop immediately if you have any concerns or discomfort and speak with your healthcare team.

Aerobic exercise

The increasing size and weight of your bump is likely to dictate what type of aerobic exercise you do during trimester 3. In general, all the exercises you were doing during trimester 2 are still safe to practise now, even running if you have been running throughout your pregnancy. That said, the elevated pressure on your pelvic floor during trimester 3 will likely bring to an end any serious running, together with most types of on-land jumping and bouncing exercise. You should also take care with high-impact exercise given the enforced change in posture leading to increased stress on the back and pelvis. In addition, the alterations in your balance and coordination due to the changes in your centre of gravity may make rapid changes in direction or complex choreographed exercises difficult to carry out. Combined, the increased weight on your pelvic floor, your altered posture and shifted centre of gravity tend to dictate a move away from high-impact, weight-bearing aerobic exercise such as running, step or dance classes towards low-load-bearing alternatives such as walking, swimming, cross-trainer or cycling. Rowing, while remaining safe, might become a little unwieldy given the size of your bump in this final trimester.

Water-based activities are a fabulous form of exercise during trimester 3, as the extra buoyancy can really take the weight off your feet, and your mind! Swimming continues to be an excellent aerobic exercise. Because you can easily control how hard you are working and how long you swim for, it is a great way to exercise if you have any worries about overdoing it. It is important to note that due to the ongoing effect of relaxin on your joints and the increased size of your bump, a little more care is needed with the breaststroke leg kick in trimester 3 (particularly if you are already suffering from pelvic girdle pain, PGP). Of course, if you have been working on your strength, core strength and stability throughout your pregnancy, you are less likely to have problems.

The magic RPE number 7 (75 per cent of your maximum heart rate) remains important during trimester 3 and with the increased size and weight of your bump that means you'll have to slow down a little to ensure you are not overdoing it. If working too hard is not your problem, and it is the desire *not* to exercise at all that is leading you to the sofa rather than the gym, don't worry; it is not necessary to reach an RPE of 7 in order to benefit from exercise. Listen to your body (and mind), and on days that you can't face a dedicated exercise session, don't sit down and do nothing at all; simply choose a different activity that is more interesting, social and fun! Go for a walk or a swim with friends or family. After all, a change is as good as a rest!

Anything is better than nothing! There are bound to be times during trimester 3 when you really can't face exercise. Don't despair – it is only natural as your motivation ebbs and flows throughout this final run-up to giving birth. In the meantime, be as active as you can and avoid prolonged sitting or lying. You will benefit from any activity, so keep moving. Every little helps!

Thirty minutes of exercise per day remains your goal, but during trimester 3 you may want to divide your daily workouts into more manageable 10-minute chunks. Research shows that three 10-minute sessions can be as effective as a single 30-minute bout of exercise for maintaining health and well-being. By splitting your workout into three separate bouts, you can easily choose different types of activity (particularly if you're in the gym) for each of the 10-minute sessions, which will have a positive effect on your motivation. Alternatively, you could try fartlek (see page 33) to add variety.

Of course, 30 minutes of exercise is a guideline and there is no reason why you cannot exercise for longer periods of time if you feel you are able to do so. As always, the duration of exercise you undertake in trimester 3 will be dictated by your exercise programme prior to pregnancy and during trimesters 1 and 2. Irrespective of the duration, your target RPE should still be at or below 7 or 75 per cent of your maximum heart rate, and you should avoid overheating. You must have a good understanding of how you respond to prolonged exercise, including hydration and nutrition, to ensure that you avoid running out of energy and becoming dehydrated.

As well as monitoring your RPE or heart rate, you can assess your post-exercise fatigue the day after your session. In general, if you are excessively fatigued 24 hours after your session, you should consider altering your programme. You should avoid chronic fatigue, as it will have a negative impact on your quality of life during this very important final stage of your pregnancy. As always, listen to your body and seek professional advice if you have any concerns.

The exercise cycle. Every exercise session should follow these simple steps:

- **Warm-up:** gradually increase your heart rate, breathing rate and muscle/body temperature with a progressive warm-up.
- **Flexibility:** a short stretching session (5 minutes is plenty) will prepare your joints and muscles for the session.
- **Exercise:** whether it's an aerobic or strength session, make sure you remain at or below an RPE of 7 (75 per cent of your maximum heart rate) and avoid overheating.
- **Cool-down:** don't just stop exercising instantly; think about an easy cool-down followed by a light stretch to ensure you return to a near-resting state after your session.

Top Tip: Underwater running while wearing a buoyancy vest is a fabulous way of continuing running as part of your routine if you're finding it a bit too demanding on land. As always, remember to avoid overheating (underwater running can be hard work) and stay at or below your RPE of 7 (75 per cent of your maximum heart rate).

AEROBIC EXERCISES: TRIMESTER 3

Repeat each of the exercises for 30 seconds to a minute.

Use music to dictate timing. Choose a tempo of music that you can maintain without excessive fatigue (an RPE of 7 or less, or 75 per cent or less of your maximum heart rate; see Chapter 2).

Remember, it is very important to maintain good posture throughout each exercise: draw your shoulder blades back, stand tall through your spine, draw your abdominals in slightly and tuck your pelvis under (bring your pubic bone up towards your belly button).

1 Marching

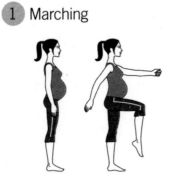

- Stand with feet shoulder-width apart with soft knees
- Draw your belly button towards your back and tighten your bum and thighs
- Lift your right knee up as high as is comfortable (maintain balance) while swinging your left arm forward
- Return to start position under control
- Repeat for your left knee

2 Side step

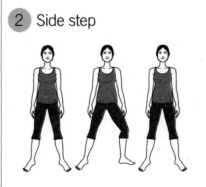

- Stand with feet shoulder-width apart with soft knees
- Draw your belly button towards your back and tighten your bum and thighs
- Step to the right with your right foot and then your left
- Step to the left (back to start position) with your left foot then your right

3 Toe tap

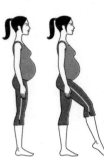

- Stand with feet shoulder-width apart with soft knees
- Draw your belly button towards your back and tighten your bum and thighs
- Lift your right leg and extend the foot forward to tap the toe on the ground directly in front
- Return to start position under control
- Repeat for your left leg

4 Heel tap

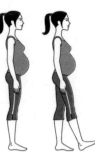

- Stand with feet shoulder-width apart with soft knees
- Draw your belly button towards your back and tighten your bum and thighs
- Lift your right leg and extend the foot forward to tap the heel on the ground directly in front
- Return to start position under control
- Repeat for your left leg

5 Arm swing

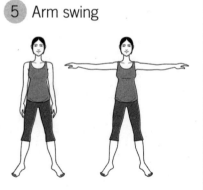

- Stand with feet shoulder-width apart with soft knees
- Draw your belly button towards your back and tighten your bum and thighs
- Swing both arms out sideways to shoulder height
- Return to start position under control

6 Squat

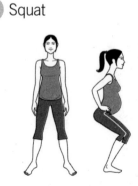

- Stand with feet shoulder-width apart with soft knees
- Draw your belly button towards your back and tighten your bum and thighs
- Bend both legs to a maximum of 90° (use a chair to touch your bottom on if you're unsure where to stop)
- Return to start position under control

7 Knee lift

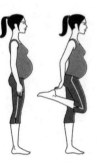

- Stand with feet shoulder-width apart with soft knees
- Draw your belly button towards your back and tighten your bum and thighs
- Lift your right knee up as high as is comfortable (maintain balance)
- Return to start position under control
- Repeat for your left knee

8 Feet to bum

- Stand with feet shoulder-width apart with soft knees
- Draw your belly button towards your back and tighten your bum and thighs
- Lift your right heel up to touch your bottom
- Return to start position under control
- Repeat for your left heel

9 Side swing

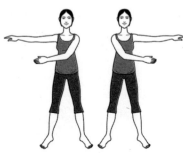

- Stand with feet shoulder-width apart with soft knees
- Draw your belly button towards your back and tighten your bum and thighs
- Swing both arms towards the right
- Return to start position under control
- Repeat to the left

10 Sumo squat

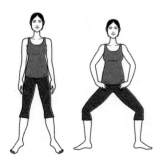

- Stand with feet wider than shoulder-width apart (as wide as you feel comfortable) with soft knees
- Draw your belly button towards your back and tighten your bum and thighs
- Keeping your back straight, head up and looking forwards, bend both legs to a maximum of 90° (use a chair to touch your bottom on if you're unsure where to stop)
- Return to start position under control

Strength exercise

This form of exercise does what it says on the tin – it promotes strength. To that end, it remains important during trimester 3 that you use a flexible band or weights to increase resistance to build/maintain strength. However, given the increased size and weight of your bump, the change in your posture and altered balance and coordination, you should ensure you modify the exercises, including reducing the weight you lift, to remain safe.

> **Top Tip:** Concentrate on technique and maintain control throughout your strength exercises; never rush or make sudden and rapid changes in direction. Concentrate on your breathing by slowly exhaling during contractions and do not hold your breath.

Given the increased stress on your back, hips and abdominals, it is increasingly important throughout this trimester to maintain good posture and good technique during exercise. Reduce the weight, the reps and/or the sets if you feel that your technique is deteriorating.

The same exercises you used in trimester 2 remain safe during trimester 3, but you should consider adapting them in line with your altered balance and coordination; for example, using a wall to lean against or a chair to hold on to while lifting can provide you with the stability and peace of mind to exercise safely. Machine weights might be a nice alternative, offering built-in stability. However, make sure you seek expert advice if you are new to the plethora of machines on offer.

The same rules for trimester 2 apply to strength exercise in trimester 3:

- Avoid exercises lying on your back or your tummy.
- Avoid exercises that directly work your abdominals.

- Avoid exercises that require rapid twisting or rapid changes in direction.
- Avoid an excessive range of motion.

Moving backwards is going in the right direction. As you progress through your pregnancy, the variety of classes on offer can remain a central part of your exercise programme. The key is to recognize your limitations when it comes to intensity, balance and coordination. Rather than give up on classes, think about moving from advanced classes to intermediate to beginner as your pregnancy progresses. Moving to lower-intensity, less complex classes means you can keep doing the exercise you love safely.

STRENGTH AND TONE: TRIMESTER 3

During your third trimester you can complete the following exercises without resistance, i.e. weights or band; however, if you do choose to use weights make sure that you are exercising within your intensity limits (RPE of 7 or below). The resistance you choose (weights or band) is likely to be different for each exercise and only consider increasing the resistance when you can easily complete all repetitions.

Always complete the exercises slowly and under control. Rest for around 1 minute between exercises. Remember to keep your RPE at 7 or below, avoid overheating and have fluid with you to drink when required.

1 Squat

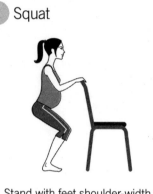

- Stand with feet shoulder-width apart, holding on to a chair for stability if required
- Draw your belly button towards your back and tighten your bum and thighs
- Keeping your back straight, head up and looking forwards, bend your legs to 90°
- Return to start position and repeat 20 times

2 Sumo squat

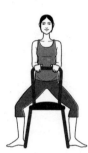

- Stand with legs just more than shoulder-width apart with feet turned out, holding on to a chair for stability if required
- Draw your belly button towards your back and tighten your bum and thighs
- Squat down, keeping your back straight and looking forwards
- Return to start position and repeat 20 times

3 Lunge

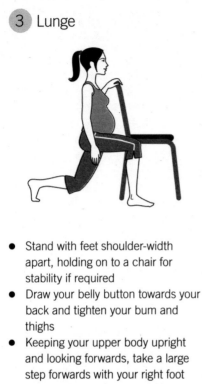

- Stand with feet shoulder-width apart, holding on to a chair for stability if required
- Draw your belly button towards your back and tighten your bum and thighs
- Keeping your upper body upright and looking forwards, take a large step forwards with your right foot and bend your front leg to 90°, keeping your knee over your foot
- Return to start position
- Repeat for your left leg
- Repeat 10 times

4 Knee lift

- Stand with feet shoulder-width apart with soft knees, holding on to a chair for stability if required
- Draw your belly button towards your back and tighten your bum and thighs
- Lift your right knee up as high as is comfortable (maintain balance)
- Return to start position under control
- Repeat for your left knee
- Repeat 10 times

5 Side arm lift

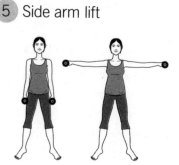

- Stand with feet shoulder-width apart with soft knees, palms facing the sides of your thighs
- Keep your back straight, head up and look forwards
- Draw your belly button towards your back and tighten your bum and thighs
- Keeping the arms straight, raise both arms out to the side until they are level with your shoulders
- Return to start position and repeat 20 times

6 Front arm lift

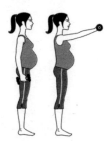

- Stand with feet shoulder-width apart with soft knees, palms facing the side of your thighs
- Keep your back straight, head up and look forwards
- Draw your belly button towards your back and tighten your bum and thighs
- Keeping the arms straight, raise them both directly in front of you until they are roughly level with your shoulders
- Return to start position and repeat 20 times

7 Prayer

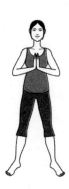

- Stand with feet shoulder-width apart with soft knees
- In front of your chest, place the palms of your hands together in a prayer-like pose
- Draw your belly button towards your back and tighten your bum and thighs
- Squeeze your hands together firmly and hold for 10 seconds
- Relax and repeat 10 times

Core strength and stability

Maintaining the strength of the postural muscles of your trunk and spine becomes increasingly important during trimester 3. Making sure you look after your core, pelvic floor and back and shoulder strength will improve your posture and reduce the likelihood of back pain and pelvic pain (often called pelvic girdle pain or PGP).

As with all types of exercise in trimester 3, you will need to think about modifying some exercises and avoiding others. If you prefer classes such as Pilates, try to find a session dedicated to pregnancy or, if none are available, think about moving down a class from intermediate to beginner to make sure you are not working beyond your capabilities. (Having an instructor qualified and experienced in prenatal exercise is of real value.)

Top Tips

- Avoid exercises that involve lying on your back or tummy.
- Avoid exercises that directly work your abdominal muscles.
- Avoid 'doming' your abdominal muscles (don't allow your tummy to be stretched outwards).
- Reduce the period of time you hold contractions.
- Breathe during contractions; do not hold your breath.
- Increase the period of recovery between exercises.
- Take care moving down to and getting up from the floor and changing positions.
- Divide your sessions into shorter periods if you are finding them too long.
- Keep your movements slow and controlled.
- Listen to your body and work at your own pace.

If it hasn't already done so, it is very likely that your *linea alba* (the connective tissue between your abdominal muscles) will begin to split during trimester 3 as the growth of your bump accelerates. The message from trimester 2 remains the same for trimester 3: 'mind the gap'. It is increasingly important that you avoid exercises that directly work the abdominals. Core strength and stability exercises on all fours are ideal during trimester 3.

Core strength and stability exercises often provide you with the time, space and peace for relaxation and ease the stresses of life. A light session before bedtime can help promote sleep and improve sleep quality.

Stand up straight!

Carrying your ever-growing bump and breasts means maintaining good posture is crucial if you are to limit the possibility of back and neck pain. In addition, the occasional headaches that are common during pregnancy are often due to stress in your upper back and neck related to poor posture. Remember, good posture is not limited to standing; you should focus on good posture when sitting and even when sleeping. To improve your posture at night, consider using pillows under your bump, between your legs and behind your back. In addition, make sure you have the right pillow supporting your head. You may need to experiment with different combinations of pillows until you find the right support for you. For sitting, here are a few ideas to help improve your posture and reduce back pain:

- Sit up with your back straight and your shoulders back. Your bum should touch the back of your chair.
- Avoid slumping and consider support for your lumbar (lower back).
- Sit with your weight distributed evenly between both bum cheeks (avoid leaning).

- Make sure your feet are flat on the floor. If your chair is too high, use a footrest that lets you rest your feet at a level that's comfortable. Your feet should be slightly lower than your hips.
- Avoid crossing your legs. (This may already be a physical impossibility due to the size of your bump!)
- Avoid sitting in the same position for more than 30 minutes; move regularly.
- When standing up, move to the front of your chair and stand up by straightening your legs. Avoid bending forward at your waist.

Flexibility

You should be stretching throughout your pregnancy either as part of your warm-up and cool-down or in dedicated sessions to maintain your flexibility and reduce tension and pain in your muscles and joints. In trimester 3, flexibility remains an important part of your exercise programme but keep in mind the changes that are taking place in your body to ensure you don't over-stretch yourself (no pun intended!). The hormone relaxin, which peaked at 12 weeks, will begin to increase again towards the end of trimester 3. The softening of ligaments around the joints means that you will be able to get into positions that were previously beyond your reach. It is important that you do not over-stretch with your new-found flexibility and focus on maintaining your range of motion rather than trying to improve it. Now is not the time to become a gymnast! The following are important guidelines for stretching during trimester 3.

- Avoid lying on your back or tummy to stretch.
- Stretch to the point where you feel your muscles lengthening and hold (10 to 30 seconds is a good target for the hold).
- Do not stretch to your maximum; if it's painful, it's too far!

- Breathe normally; do not hold your breath.
- Ensure you are stable and in full control during the stretch (use support if required).
- Avoid abdominal stretches, touching toes (seated or standing), wide leg stretches such as the splits or hurdle stretch particularly if you have pelvic pain, dynamic (bouncing) stretching and excessive range of motion in any stretch.

Stretch it out! It is not uncommon to feel too tired to exercise during the third trimester. However, a gentle flexibility session can help ease those aches and pains without too much effort. In addition, completing a session will make you feel like you are doing something positive to help yourself, which will make you feel a whole lot better.

CORE STRENGTH AND STABILITY: TRIMESTER 3

1 Abdominal hollowing

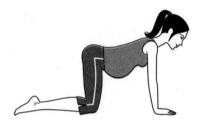

- Start on all fours with your weight evenly distributed between hands and knees and your back long and straight
- Breathe out and relax your abdominals
- Breathing in, slowly squeeze in your abdominals (do not squeeze too hard and ensure you can breathe at all times)
- Return to start position and repeat 10 times

2 Cat and extension

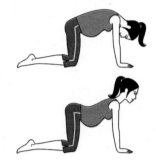

- Start on all fours with your weight evenly distributed
- Draw your belly button towards your back and tense your legs and bottom
- Allowing your head to drop, slowly arch your back upwards and hold momentarily
- Return to start position
- Without doming your abdominals, lift your head and slowly arch your back to the floor and hold momentarily
- Return to start position and repeat 10 times

3 All fours with arm lift

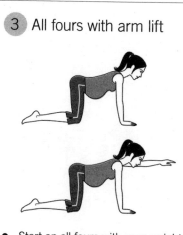

- Start on all fours with your weight evenly distributed and your back long and straight
- Draw your belly button towards your back and tense your legs and bottom
- Without collapsing your right arm, extend your left arm directly forwards
- Hold for 10 seconds
- Return to start position
- Repeat for your right arm
- Relax and repeat 5 times

4 All fours with leg lift

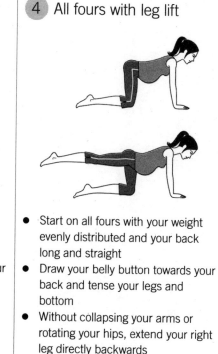

- Start on all fours with your weight evenly distributed and your back long and straight
- Draw your belly button towards your back and tense your legs and bottom
- Without collapsing your arms or rotating your hips, extend your right leg directly backwards
- Hold for 10 seconds
- Return to start position
- Repeat for your left leg
- Relax and repeat 5 times

5 Superwoman

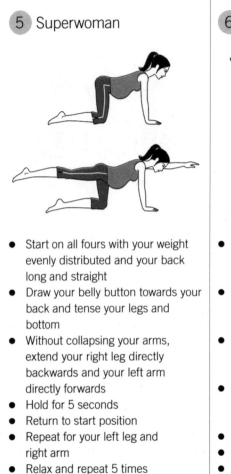

- Start on all fours with your weight evenly distributed and your back long and straight
- Draw your belly button towards your back and tense your legs and bottom
- Without collapsing your arms, extend your right leg directly backwards and your left arm directly forwards
- Hold for 5 seconds
- Return to start position
- Repeat for your left leg and right arm
- Relax and repeat 5 times

6 Thread the needle

- Start on all fours with your weight evenly distributed and your back long and straight
- Draw your belly button towards your back and tense your legs and bottom
- Without collapsing your arms, extend your right arm to the side directly above you
- Under control, move your right arm under your body as far as you can to the left
- Return to start position
- Repeat for your left arm
- Relax and repeat 5 times

BUMP IT UP

Side plank

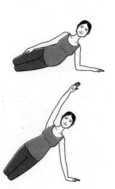

- Sit on your left hip with your legs bent at the knee, resting on your left elbow
- Draw your belly button towards your back and tense your legs and bottom
- Keeping your weight through your knees and without collapsing your arm, lift your hips, making a straight line from shoulder to hip to knee
- Return to start position and repeat 10 times
- Roll over and repeat for your right hip

8 **Side kick**

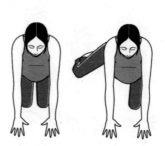

- Start on all fours with your weight evenly distributed and your back long and straight
- Draw your belly button towards your back and tense your legs and bottom
- Without collapsing your arms or rotating your hips, lift your right knee out to the side as far as you can
- Return to start position
- Repeat for your left leg
- Relax and repeat 10 times

9 All fours with reverse toe touch

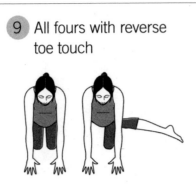

- Start on all fours with your weight evenly distributed and your back long and straight
- Draw your belly button towards your back and tense your legs and bottom
- Without collapsing your arms, extend your right leg to the side and touch your toe on the ground as far to the left side of your body as you can
- Return to start position
- Repeat for your left leg
- Relax and repeat 10 times

10 Side leg raise

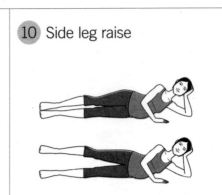

- Lie on your left side with your left arm bent at the elbow to support your head and your right arm in front of you supporting your body
- Draw your belly button towards your back and tense your legs and bottom
- Straighten your body and, without falling forwards or backwards, lift your right leg by about 15cm, keeping the leg straight
- Return to start position and repeat 10 times
- Roll over and repeat for your left leg

You guessed it, pelvic floor exercises! I know it might seem a bit repetitious but if it's worth saying once it's worth repeating for pre-pregnancy, trimesters 1 to 3 and even post-partum. If ever there was a time for pelvic floor exercises, trimester 3 is it. So if you do nothing else, make sure you continue with your pelvic floor exercises.

The exercise programme for trimester 3

As your bump grows, so too does the importance of exercise during trimester 3. Although you may feel less and less like exercising as you enter the final stretch, it is exactly because this is the trimester where the greatest stretch and weight increase occurs that you need to ensure you stay on top of your physical well-being. Do remember, your exercise programme is not set in stone. Remain flexible by taking advantage of those days when you feel like exercising, and modifying exercise on those days when you are just too tired. The only caveat to this flexible approach is to make sure you always do something, even if it is only an easy walk or a light stretch. And at the risk of sounding boring, don't forget your daily pelvic floor exercises!

The same general guidelines for exercise from trimesters 1 and 2 remain, but modification is the key word in trimester 3. Rather than tackling your exercise programme all in one bite, consider grazing – splitting your sessions into smaller, more manageable chunks. You will gain similar benefits but put less pressure on yourself both physically and emotionally.

For aerobic exercise, think about using an interval or fartlek structure to break up the intensity. With your growing bump, it is also time to consider lower-load-bearing activities such as swimming, aquarobics and cycling.

When it comes to strength exercises, the main change is a

reduction in resistance – the weight you are lifting. As ever, an RPE of 7 (75 per cent of your maximum heart rate) remains the upper end of your intensity target, but remember anything is better than nothing, so don't let working to this limit stand in your way of activity.

The more active you remain through trimester 3, the better able you are to cope with the inevitable aches and pains that accompany your growing bump. Importantly, the better your aerobic capacity, strength, core strength and stability, pelvic floor strength, and flexibility, the more prepared you will be for delivery and the quicker you will return to full fitness post-partum.

EXERCISE IN TRIMESTER 3

Aerobic:	30 minutes at least 5 days per week (split into 10-minute bouts spread across the day or try fartlek or interval exercise)
Strength:	1 to 2 sessions per week (30 minutes in duration or you could try shorter sessions more frequently, i.e. multiple 10-minute sessions spread across the week)
Core strength and stability:	2 to 3 sessions per week
Pelvic floor:	daily

Trimester 3 FAQs

Why do I waddle like a duck?

Your posture is likely to change during trimester 3 as you adapt to the increased size and weight of your bump. It is not uncommon to walk with your feet slightly wider apart, which in turn will cause the hips to drop alternately on each step, resulting in that characteristic waddling movement. The additional downside to looking like Daffy Duck is the extra stress this movement places on your back, hips and knees, leading to instability and pain (remember your joints are that little laxer due to the circulating relaxin). It is important to strengthen your core, bum and legs to reduce/eliminate the waddle. You will be thankful for the extra effort you put in in the long run.

Can I start strength exercise in the third trimester?

You can begin exercising at any time during your pregnancy and benefit from all the positive effects associated with a more active life-style. When it comes to strength training, the same rules apply as with any new exercise or return to exercise:

- Make sure you begin gently (one set of each exercise will be enough at the beginning).
- Increase intensity slowly (start with low or no weight at an RPE of 4 and increase the weight up to an RPE of 7 over time).
- Listen to your body, stop if you have any concerns and speak to your healthcare team.

There are a couple of caveats I would add in relation to starting your strength training in trimester 3:

- Speak with your healthcare team before starting strength exercise to ensure it is safe to do so.
- Seek the advice and support of an appropriately qualified personal trainer to make sure you use the appropriate weights and technique.

Can I do yoga in trimester 3?

Yoga is generally safe across all three trimesters. However, as with all aspects of your exercise programme you will need to adapt your sessions in line with your stage of pregnancy as well as your physical condition and experience.

If you are thinking about starting yoga for the first time in trimester 3, make sure you speak with your healthcare team and find a complete beginners class taught by a qualified and experienced teacher.

In addition to the physical benefits of improved/maintained flexibility and stability, yoga provides a wonderful opportunity for a break from the hustle and bustle of daily living. Escaping the world outside provides a time for mindfulness and relaxation.

There are some forms of yoga that should be avoided. Dynamic yoga should not be practised unless you are very experienced, and even experienced yoga enthusiasts may want to think carefully about dynamic yoga in trimester 3! Bikram yoga is definitely one to avoid throughout pregnancy due to the increased risk of overheating.

Will exercise cause premature delivery of my baby?

There is no evidence to suggest that moderate-intensity exercise at any stage during pregnancy leads to pre-term delivery in low-risk pregnancies. Indeed, recent evidence suggests that women who exercise regularly throughout pregnancy are less likely to require a caesarean section.

PREGNANCY TRIVIA

It's a boy!

If you're having a little boy, it's not until month 8 that his testicles will move into the sac specifically designed to house them: the scrotum. Around 4 per cent of boys will be born with non-descended testicles, but they usually drop within the first year.

Seeing is believing

By the end of month 7, your baby will not only be able to blink but their irises will respond to changes in light by contracting. This also allows them to focus on objects, although they won't use this skill until they are in the outside world.

Immunity from disease

Your baby's immune system is developing rapidly during trimester 3. However, your baby will rely on you to provide antibodies through the placenta to help protect it from infection. Even after birth, you continue to provide support to their immune system through the delivery of antibodies in your breast milk.

Breath of life

One of the important developments in your baby's lungs occurs in trimester 3 with the production of surfactant. This phospholipoprotein (a big word for a complex with a combination of fats and proteins) acts to create surface tension in the small sacs in the lungs called alveoli (the place where we uptake oxygen and remove carbon dioxide). Without this the alveoli would not stay open and the lungs would not be able to function in the outside world.

It's never too late

You can begin exercising at any stage of pregnancy, so never think you've left it too late. As long as you remember to start easy and progress slowly, listening to your body throughout, and remain at or below an RPE of 7 (75 per cent of your maximum heart rate), you'll be able to enjoy the benefits of exercise whenever you start. And if nothing else, you can do your pelvic floor exercises anywhere and at any time. You won't even have to stand up if you don't want to!

Relax

Levels of the hormone relaxin peak at around 12 to 14 weeks and again towards the end of pregnancy as you approach the birth of your baby. The release of relaxin in the final stages of pregnancy not only helps in the growth, opening and softening of the cervix and vagina to aid birth, it also promotes the breaking of the membrane that surrounds the baby prior to birth. Believe it or not, men produce relaxin in their testes! While the role of relaxin is not clear in men, it may be associated with improving the motility of sperm.

6

Post–Partum: Birth to 6 Weeks

CONGRATULATIONS! You're a mum – and perhaps not for the first time! Having successfully dealt with pregnancy and the delivery of your new baby, you must now, simultaneously, deal with the task of becoming a new mum and the huge changes that have taken place and which continue to occur in your body. While your new addition absorbs most of the attention in this post-partum period, and beyond, it is crucial that you also maintain a focus on YOU.

All too often the delivery of your baby is seen as the end point of the high-quality care you, and others, have taken of your well-being. However, the World Health Organization (WHO) considers the post-partum period to be the most critical and yet the most neglected phase in the lives of mothers. So putting your new baby first does not have to mean that you are suddenly relegated to the sidelines; how healthy and happy you are will have a direct impact on your baby.

Immediately after birth, your uterus weighs around 1kg, but will rapidly reduce in size and weight to only 2oz by the end of the post-partum period. Within a few days of delivery, your breasts will become engorged as your milk production accelerates; this often leads to very tender breasts and the leaking of milk. After vaginal births, the pressure placed on your bladder during delivery can result in difficulty urinating, together with a burning sensation. Urinary and even faecal incontinence is not uncommon following vaginal delivery and is primarily associated with weakness in your pelvic floor muscles. While this can be embarrassing, it will reverse in time and this will happen even more rapidly if you strengthen your pelvic floor muscles.

The delivery of a baby is a major physical trauma, whether you have given birth vaginally or via caesarean section (C-section). In addition, the psychological effort of childbirth, combined with hormonal changes and your new responsibilities as a mother, can often result in significant emotional upheaval during the post-partum period. While many of these changes may normalize relatively quickly (in a matter of weeks), some, including emotional and psychological fluctuations, may persist over longer periods.

Following childbirth, the levels of the hormones oestrogen and progesterone, which steadily increased during pregnancy, fall sharply, reaching pre-pregnancy levels around five days after delivery. Levels of hormones produced by your thyroid gland also fall, along with those of other hormones such as human chorionic gonadotropin (HCG). These rapid and dramatic changes in your hormones, together with the effort of childbirth and coping with your new arrival, can result in fatigue, lethargy and, for some new mums, depression.

Soon after delivery, it is also not uncommon to experience hair loss. Rather than this being a true loss of hair, this process is simply a normalization of your scalp as, due to hormonal changes, you retained hair during pregnancy that you would normally have lost. So after delivery, you may start losing more hair than normal and this process may last for up to six months post-partum.

Changes in skin pigmentation that might have occurred during pregnancy, for example a brown line down the centre of your tummy, should now begin to disappear. In contrast, stretch marks, together with the additional weight around your tummy (often loose and flabby skin), will take longer to reverse. Again, focused exercise and a healthy diet will accelerate the return to your pre-pregnancy weight and shape.

What changes can I expect in the post-partum period?

You have delivered your baby and in the following weeks you will experience a different set of changes, with the first six weeks post-partum considered the recovery period. It is important to listen carefully to your body, and your healthcare team, during this time to ensure you optimize your return to normal life – although 'normal' life will never be quite the same again!

Your body has undergone a nine-month-long evolution, which has been topped off with one of the most physical and emotional efforts of your life – more than any man ever experiences! During that time, your body has been pulled, pushed and stretched, your hormones have been constantly changing, and your emotions have been on a rollercoaster ride since conception. Accordingly, it will take time to readjust physically and mentally. You can't force a return to normality, but you can make sure you do the right things to help support a speedy recovery.

As with your entire pregnancy, the individuality of the post-partum period means that you may experience some, none or all of the changes mentioned. Indeed, you may have other less common symptoms that are not reported in books, magazines or online. It is important to remember that if you have any concerns at all, speak with your healthcare professional. Overleaf are common changes during the six-week post-partum recovery period:

PHYSICAL AND EMOTIONAL CHANGES: POST-PARTUM PERIOD

	Vaginal birth	C-section	Reducing over the six-week recovery period
PHYSICAL			
Fatigue	✓ likely to be exhausted for a week or so	✓ the same or less than vaginal depending on the period of labour	✓
General aches and pains all over your body from pushing	✓		✓
Vaginal bleeding (termed 'lochia', mimicking your period – a combination of blood, mucus and uterine tissue leads to colour changes from dark red initially to brownish to yellowish)	✓	✓	✓ changing
Vaginal cramps	✓	✓	✓
Stomach pain associated with shrinking uterus	✓	✓	✓
Perineal discomfort (including pain and numbness)	✓ greater discomfort following episiotomy or tearing	✓ minimal, dependent on duration of labour	✓

	Vaginal birth	C-section	Reducing over the six-week recovery period
Wound pain		✓	✓ evolving from pain to numbness
Haemorrhoids (continued from pregnancy or new from the effort of pushing during labour)	✓	✓	✓
Difficulty/discomfort going to the toilet (for urination or defecation)	✓	✓	✓
Breast engorgement and discomfort	✓	✓	✓
Discomfort when walking due to wound repair	✓ episiotomy or tearing	✓	✓
Back and pelvic pain (and general joint pain from relaxin-related increased laxity during pregnancy)	✓	✓	✓
Reduced weight and swelling	✓	✓	✓
Poor sleep quality	✓	✓	✓
Excessive sweating	✓	✓	✓
Hair loss	✓	✓	✓
EMOTIONAL			
Mood swings, irritability, irrationality, unexpected crying (heightened premenstrual syndrome) associated with hormone changes	✓	✓	✓
Excitement, anxiety, fear, feeling overwhelmed	✓	✓	✓

Exercise and the post-partum period

Being active after giving birth plays a key role in your recovery and your return to full health in a variety of ways. The 'feel-good factor' of exercise can help improve mood and, combined with an improvement in strength, stamina and mobility, can help you cope with becoming a new mum. Exercise, together with a healthy, well-balanced diet can also help you take a positive, proactive approach to managing your weight while ensuring you provide the right nutrients to optimize the healing process and recovery from the exertion of labour and childbirth. It can sometimes feel a bit counterintuitive to exercise when you feel more exhausted than at any other time in your life, but exercise can actually invigorate you and reduce the feeling of tiredness. In addition, with sleep often in short supply with a newborn, returning to regular exercise can help improve your quality of sleep.

When should you start?

There's no time like the present! Exercise can begin almost immediately after birth. In fact, getting mobile again is an important part of reducing the risk of some complications during the immediate post-partum period and should be encouraged where possible. You don't even have to stand up to start making a difference; you can start working those pelvic floor muscles in the first 24 hours after delivery! But one word of warning: although you can begin soon after delivery, make sure you take it nice and slowly at first, gradually building up your exercise regime. As always, listen carefully to your body.

What exercises should I target first?

In the early post-partum period, pelvic floor muscle exercises are important to help stabilize your pelvic floor, improve control and reduce incontinence. Pelvic floor exercises can also speed up the rate of healing following tearing or an episiotomy. You can also start tummy exercises, but make sure you introduce them gradually, giving yourself time to recover between efforts (see page 161 for the differences between vaginal and C-section births). Split abdominals, or diastasis (see page 63), are a common problem and there are a range of exercises you can do to 'close the gap'. In addition to the tummy area, make sure you strengthen your back. The impact of pregnancy and childbirth, combined with an instantaneous change in your centre of gravity post-delivery and poor posture during feeding and carrying your new baby, can lead to lower- and upper-back problems. Making sure you focus on these areas can improve your posture and reduce pain and discomfort.

Due in part to hormonal changes, it is very common to feel emotional, anxious and a little down following childbirth – so common, in fact, that these feelings are often called the 'baby blues'. The baby blues do not usually last for more than two weeks after delivery. However, if these symptoms persist, or begin later in the post-partum period, it is likely that you are suffering from postnatal depression (PND). If you feel that you may be suffering from PND, you should speak to your healthcare adviser immediately. They can offer you the support and advice you need during this difficult period. And remember, exercise can be very helpful in reducing the symptoms of PND and improving your general outlook. Research has shown that postnatal exercise classes can be particularly successful, as exercise can be combined with the sharing of experiences and can create a sense of community.

Getting back to activity doesn't have to be a solo endeavour. Exercising with your baby has been shown to improve the mother–baby bond as well as increasing the well-being of both mother and baby. There are a range of exercise options that include mother and baby, but one of my favourites is swimming, with a number of organizations now providing mother and baby classes (check out www.turtletots.com, for example). Importantly, these are not just mother-and-baby organizations; fathers can, and should, get involved too!

Top Tips:

- Be as active as possible following delivery (pelvic floor and ab work can start within 24 hours).
- Start very slowly and progress at a comfortable and achievable rate.
- Dividing your exercise up into small packages can make it much more achievable and productive.
- Perform exercise slowly so that you remain in full control.
- Your joints remain lax after birth, so take care with rapid, jerky movements and don't over-stretch.
- Listen to your body and make adjustments as necessary; your programme is not set in stone!

BENEFITS OF EXERCISE IN THE POST-PARTUM PERIOD:

- reduces post-delivery complications
- supports healing and accelerates recovery from labour and delivery
- improves mental and emotional well-being
- reduces back and neck pain
- improves pelvic floor muscles and reduces incontinence
- stabilizes lax joints
- reduces a range of post-partum symptoms from leg cramps to sexual problems
- improves sleep
- boosts energy levels and reduces fatigue
- improves quality of life

Aerobic exercise

Aerobic activity should remain central to your exercise programme during the post-partum period. While you may not feel up to formal exercise sessions at this time, it is important that you are as active as possible. Invariably, this means walking in the days and first few weeks following delivery, which is perfect to support your return to full fitness and health. Walking is a wonderfully social activity post-partum that you can share with your baby (pushing their buggy or carrying them) and your family and friends. Take it slowly at the start, only walking for short periods of time, interspersed with rest. You can choose to walk short routes or, alternatively, plan walks where you know there are benches – or coffee shops – where you can stop to recover and refuel! As you begin to feel more comfortable and confident, gradually increase the distance you walk. Although the target remains at 30 minutes per day, you can divide your walking into shorter packages spread across the day.

How intensively should I exercise in the post-partum period?

The intensity of exercise is very much an individual matter during the post-partum period and much less precise when compared with the three trimesters of pregnancy. No longer is 7 the magic number! How hard you exercise is entirely related to how well you are coping in the days and weeks following delivery. In general, however, remember that the post-partum period is called recovery for a reason and you should structure your exercise to optimize the recovery process.

It is wise to begin your exercise at a very light/easy intensity – RPE of 3 to 5 – before beginning to increase to your pre-delivery intensity of moderate – RPE of 7. It is unlikely that you will be exercising at high intensity during the post-partum period but there is no reason why you can't if you feel able to do so. The issues related to the health of your baby, such as overheating, no longer exist. However, take care not to push too hard, too soon. As always, your level of conditioning prior to delivery will dictate how rapidly you are able to return to high-intensity exercise but, even for the fittest of new mums, it is likely to be beyond the six-week post-partum period.

When it comes to high-impact exercise, such as running and high-impact classes, it again depends on your level of conditioning prior to delivery and how well you are recovering post-delivery. In general, it is important, even for the fittest of new mums, to ensure that your pelvic floor muscles, core (including back) and joints are strong before starting any exercise that loads the joints or involves jumping or bouncing activities. When you do return to this type of exercise, which is, at the earliest, likely to be towards the end of the post-partum period, you should do so progressively. Again, listen to your body and adapt your programme accordingly.

Low-load-bearing exercises, such as walking, cross-trainer and cycling (when you can sit on the saddle), are great forms of aerobic exercise.

Swimming is a fabulous activity in the post-partum period. However, there are a number of reasons why you may not be able to start immediately, including your lochia flow (the post-delivery bleeding and discharge) and wound healing from tears, an episiotomy and/or a C-section. In contrast, your baby can go swimming at any time after birth and this is a good opportunity for partners to step in and take an active role in parenting the newborn. There is no need to wait for your baby to complete their course of vaccinations, although most parent-and-baby swimming classes do not start until a baby is six weeks old, which is around the time that you may feel ready to take the plunge.

A couple of weeks after birth, you may feel ready to progress to more formal aerobic exercise sessions. It is unlikely that this will include traditional classes, although there are now a range of early postnatal exercise groups that can add a layer of security and confidence to your return to exercise, as well as some fun and enjoyment. If you don't feel up to taking on exercise classes in these early post-partum days, here is a simple aerobic exercise programme that you can do at home. Remember, take it easy at first and gradually build your activity as your fitness and confidence grows.

AEROBIC EXERCISES: POST-PARTUM

You can complete these exercises with or without weights. If you choose to use dumbbells, you should select a weight with which you can complete all the repetitions of each exercise. Use the same weight throughout and consider increasing the weight of your dumbbells when you can complete all the exercises easily.

Repeat each of the exercises for 30 seconds to a minute, using music to help with timing. Choose a tempo of music that you can maintain throughout the session. Move through the exercises at your own pace but without resting between them. No need to stick to an RPE of 7 now; simply work as hard as you can. Remember, it is very important to maintain good posture throughout each exercise: draw your shoulder blades back, stand tall through your spine, draw your abdominals in slightly and tuck your pelvis under (bring your pubic bone up towards your belly button).

To add variety, you could choose aerobic exercises from any of the previous chapters.

1 Squat

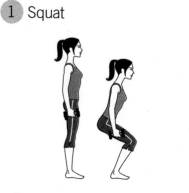

- Stand with feet shoulder-width apart and hands at the side of your thighs
- Draw your belly button towards your back and tighten your bum and thighs
- Keeping your back straight, head up and looking forwards, bend your legs to 90°
- Return to start position

2 Side step and squat

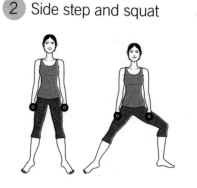

- Stand with feet shoulder-width apart and hands at the side of your thighs
- Draw your belly button towards your back and tighten your bum and thighs
- Keeping your back straight, head up and looking forwards, take a large step to your right
- Bend your left knee to 90°
- Return to start position and repeat for your left leg

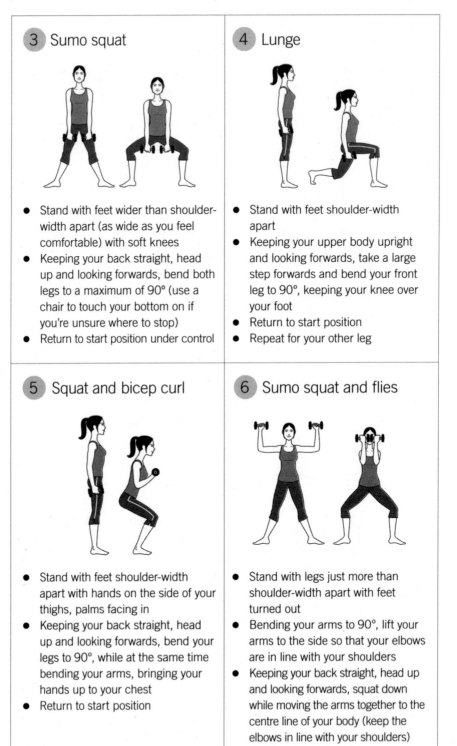

3 Sumo squat

- Stand with feet wider than shoulder-width apart (as wide as you feel comfortable) with soft knees
- Keeping your back straight, head up and looking forwards, bend both legs to a maximum of 90° (use a chair to touch your bottom on if you're unsure where to stop)
- Return to start position under control

4 Lunge

- Stand with feet shoulder-width apart
- Keeping your upper body upright and looking forwards, take a large step forwards and bend your front leg to 90°, keeping your knee over your foot
- Return to start position
- Repeat for your other leg

5 Squat and bicep curl

- Stand with feet shoulder-width apart with hands on the side of your thighs, palms facing in
- Keeping your back straight, head up and looking forwards, bend your legs to 90°, while at the same time bending your arms, bringing your hands up to your chest
- Return to start position

6 Sumo squat and flies

- Stand with legs just more than shoulder-width apart with feet turned out
- Bending your arms to 90°, lift your arms to the side so that your elbows are in line with your shoulders
- Keeping your back straight, head up and looking forwards, squat down while moving the arms together to the centre line of your body (keep the elbows in line with your shoulders)
- Return to start position

7 Knee lift and swing

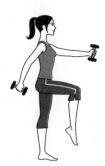

- Stand with feet shoulder-width apart with soft knees
- Keeping your back straight, head up and looking forwards, lift your right knee up as high as is comfortable (maintain balance) while swinging the left arm forwards up to the level of your shoulders
- Return to start position under control
- Repeat for your left knee and right arm

8 Squat and push press

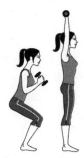

- Stand upright with feet shoulder-width apart with soft knees
- Bring your hands to your shoulders with your elbows down
- Keeping your back straight, head up and looking forwards, bend the legs to 90°
- As you stand, extend both arms upwards above your head until they are straight
- Return to start position

9 Twists

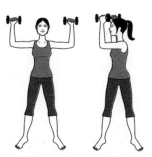

- Stand upright with feet shoulder-width apart with soft knees
- Draw your belly button towards your back and tense your legs and bottom
- Bend your arms to 90° and lift your arms to the side until your elbows are level with your shoulders
- Keeping your back straight and head up, rotate around to your right
- Return to start position and repeat, rotating around to your left

Core strength and stability

Whether you have given birth vaginally or by C-section, you won't be returning to traditional core strength and stability exercises instantly. It will take some time for your core muscles and pelvic floor to recover following delivery. Because of this, you should begin strengthening your pelvic floor and core slowly and carefully in the first few weeks. If you have had a C-section, it may take a little longer as your scar heals and your digestive system settles.

Yes, you guessed it – pelvic floor!

Although you may not feel like it, you can begin your return to exercise within 24 hours of giving birth. I know what you're thinking, but I'm not talking about running a marathon! Pelvic floor exercises (yes, that old chestnut!) can begin soon after birth and although you may not be able to feel your pelvic floor muscles due to perineal numbness (particularly if you've had an anaesthetic for an episiotomy or tearing), you can start to improve the strength of your pelvic floor almost instantly.

Pelvic floor exercises

Slow-twitch pelvic floor muscles
- Sit or lie comfortably.
- Squeeze the pelvic floor muscles.
- Hold for 1 to 2 seconds and then slowly release.
- Repeat 10 times with around 5 seconds' rest between contractions.
- Once you are able to complete this, increase the duration of time you hold the contraction (work up to 10-second holds).

Fast-twitch pelvic floor muscles

- Sit or lie comfortably.
- Squeeze the pelvic floor muscles.
- Hold for 1 second and then slowly release.
- Repeat 10 times with around 5 seconds' rest between contractions.

IMPORTANT: BREATHE! Do not hold your breath or tighten your stomach, buttock or thigh muscles at the same time.

Closing the gap

You may not have noticed a gap developing in your abdominal muscles but now is the time to check. The simplest way to do this is as follows:

- Lie on your back.
- Raise your head slightly with your arms extended forwards.
- Place the fingers of one hand just above your belly button.
- If you feel a gap, then you have a separation (also known as diastasis or split abs).
- Using your fingers, measure how big the gap is.
- Keep checking regularly throughout your recovery and you should feel the size of the gap decreasing.

You can begin to close the gap soon after giving birth. However, you should be careful and take a progressive approach to introducing abdominal-specific exercise; it will take some time and effort! In the very early days post-delivery, the following exercise is a safe, simple way to begin the process of closure:

Tummy pulls

- Lie on your back.
- Cross your arms across your tummy and place your hands on either side of your gap.
- Take a deep breath in.
- As you breathe out, slowly pull your belly button inwards towards your back and lift your head.
- Return to the start position, relax and repeat three to five times.
- Repeat three times daily.

As your abdominals get stronger, and when you feel ready, move on to the exercises outlined on the following pages. This is likely to be towards the end of the post-partum period and will depend on how well you are recovering as well as how much core work you were able to do pre-conception and during pregnancy.

At this time, you can also begin to work on your core strength and stability, which will support the return of your core muscles, including your abdominals, to full strength and function, as well as assisting in reducing the inevitable post-partum back and neck pain.

CORE AND SPLIT-AB WORKOUT: POST-PARTUM

1 Scooping

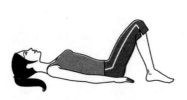

- Lie on your back, draw your belly button towards your back and tense your legs and bottom
- Hold for 5 seconds
- Repeat 10 times

2 Roll-ups

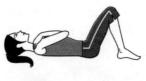

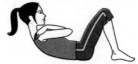

- Lying flat on your back, bend your legs with your feet on the floor
- Place your hands across your chest, touching the opposite shoulder
- Draw your belly button towards your back and tense your legs and bottom
- Pull your chin into your chest and lift your shoulders away from the floor towards your knees
- Lift your shoulders about 15cm off the floor and return slowly to the start position
- Repeat 10 times
  (Make it harder: 1) bring feet closer to bum; 2) squeeze your knees together; 3) point each elbow in turn to the opposite knee)

3 Leg kick

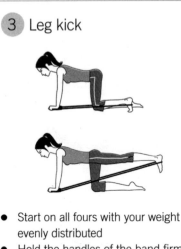

- Start on all fours with your weight evenly distributed
- Hold the handles of the band firmly in each hand and place the middle of the band on the sole of your left foot
- Draw your belly button towards your back and tense your legs and bottom
- Extend your left leg directly behind you, making a straight line between your shoulder, hip, knee and ankle
- Return to start position
- Repeat 10 times
- Repeat for your right leg

4 Clam

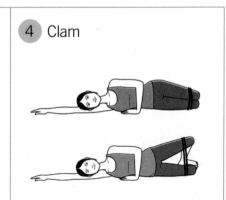

- Wrap the band securely around your knees, leaving the band loose between the knees requiring a moderate contraction to lift the knee
- Lie on your right side with your lower arm extended above your head and your upper arm in front of you supporting your body
- Keep the legs together, bent at 90°, making a straight line from your shoulders to hips to knees
- Draw your belly button towards your back
- Keeping the feet together, lift your left knee as high as possible
- Return to start position
- Repeat 20 times
- Turn over and repeat with your right leg on top

5 Cushion squeeze

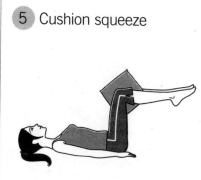

- Lie on the floor with your legs bent at 90° and place a firm cushion between your knees
- Draw your belly button towards your back and tense your legs and bottom
- Lift your legs with your thighs vertical and your lower legs parallel with the floor
- Squeeze your knees together and hold for 5 seconds
- Return to start position and repeat 20 times

6 Superwoman

- Start on all fours with your weight evenly distributed and your back long and straight
- Draw your belly button towards your back and breathe normally
- Without collapsing your left arm, extend your left leg directly backwards and your right arm directly forwards
- Hold for 5 seconds
- Return to start position
- Repeat for your right leg and left arm
- Relax and repeat 5 times

7 Plank

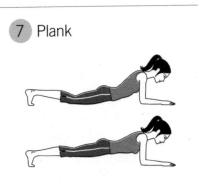

- Lie face down on the floor with your upper body supported by your forearms, elbows beneath your shoulders
- Draw your belly button towards your back and tense your legs and bottom
- Raise yourself on to your forearms and the balls of your feet, making a straight line between your heels, hips and shoulders
- Hold for 20 seconds
- Relax and repeat 5 times

8 Shoulder bridge

- Lie on your back, hands by your side and knees bent, feet shoulder-width apart
- Draw your belly button towards your back and tense your legs and bottom
- Breathe in and roll your hips to the ceiling until your are resting on your shoulders with a straight line from shoulders to hips to knees
- Hold for 10 seconds
- Return to start position and repeat 5 times

9 Toe touch

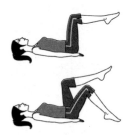

- Lie on your back with your arms by your side
- Draw your belly button towards your back and tense your legs and bottom
- Pull your knees up and hold them in the air, making a 90° angle at your hips and knees
- Contract your core and lower your right foot to the floor, touching the toe lightly on the ground before returning to the start position
- Repeat for your left leg
- Repeat 10 times

Strength exercise

Maintaining and improving your strength following the delivery of your baby is important, as it will help reduce back and neck pain, stabilize lax joints, support your return to an active lifestyle and improve your ability to cope with the activities of daily life, including carrying your baby. But during this period of recovery, you should not aim for an instantaneous return to your strength exercise programme, but rather a slow, progressive return, focusing on strength exercises for your back and core, which you can begin almost immediately after giving birth.

With careful progression, and by listening to your body, you can begin to increase your strength exercise programme across the post-partum period. As a general rule of thumb, once you are ready, use the strength exercises in Chapters 3 to 5 in reverse order, starting with the exercises from your third trimester before moving on to trimester 2 exercises and then trimester 1.

Strengthening your back

Despite the disappearance of your bump, it is not uncommon to suffer from back pain following childbirth. There are a number of reasons for this sometimes heightened pain, including the loss of abdominal muscle strength, poor posture following the instantaneous change in your centre of gravity, and carrying and breastfeeding your new baby. Exercise and ensuring correct posture are central to improving the strength and stability of your spine and reducing the pain. The pelvic tilt exercise below will help you to gently and safely strengthen your back.

Pelvic tilt exercise
- Lie on the floor with a pillow under your head.
- Pull your feet up to your bum by sliding your feet along the ground.

- Tighten your pelvic floor and abdominals.
- Squeeze the small of your lower back against the floor.
- Hold for 3 to 5 seconds, then arch your lower back to the ceiling.
- Return to start position and repeat this sequence 10 times.

Remember to breathe throughout: do not hold your breath!

TOP TIPS FOR REDUCING BACK PAIN:

- When lifting heavy objects, make sure you keep your back straight and head up. Bend from the knees and activate your legs, core and pelvic floor while lifting.
- Change nappies on an elevated surface, ensuring your baby is safe at all times. Avoid bending over your baby for prolonged periods.
- When feeding your baby, focus on your posture. Use pillows to support your back and your baby, and make sure your feet are in contact with the floor or on a stool. Avoid prolonged bending, particularly of your upper back.
- Maintain a good standing and sitting posture throughout the day, and focus on good posture during exercise.

Flexibility

While your body will reduce the production of relaxin following childbirth, the effects of the surge of relaxin pre-delivery, together with the softening of your connective tissues throughout pregnancy, means that your joints will remain lax for some time (anything up to six months). In order to avoid strain or injury, you need to remain vigilant and avoid over-stretching.

The introduction of strength exercises will begin to support your joints, helping to stabilize them over the weeks and months following delivery as your connective tissue (tendons, ligaments, etc.) begins to tighten. You should be able to complete all of the flexibility exercises from Chapter 2. Remember to go slowly and with control, and only go to the point where you feel a stretch – and then hold the stretch, rather than going further.

C-section

For mums who have had an elective or emergency C-section, there are special considerations for the post-partum period. A C-section is considered major abdominal surgery. As such, the recovery process follows the same path as for any similar surgery, but with the added burden of the usual post-partum changes for good measure! Many of the symptoms will be the same as those you might experience if you had given birth vaginally. However, additional symptoms associated with wound healing and the realignment of your digestive system, which was moved during surgery, can result in pain that can last for a number of weeks. Importantly, the trauma to your abdominal muscles means that you will need to take extra precautions when it comes to exercise. Your scar is likely to remain sore for a few weeks but will improve steadily, although you may experience numbness on and around the scar for a number of months, which is perfectly normal.

Pelvic floor exercises are still very important and, as mentioned, you can begin these soon after birth. In addition, closing the gap in your abdominal muscles and strengthening your back are the cornerstones of your return to full activity. It may take a little while longer before you feel able to introduce the tummy pulls and pelvic tilts, but don't worry, they will not rip your stitches or damage your scar. Again, listen to your body, and your healthcare team, and start when you feel ready. Recommendations for aerobic exercise are the same as those for vaginal births, and it is equally important that you are as active as possible in order to feel the benefits exercise has to offer a new mum.

The exercise programme for the post-partum period

Your bump is gone – well, almost! But the disappearance of your bump, along with all those added complications of pregnancy you have been dealing with for the last nine months, does not mean an instantaneous return to a full exercise programme.

Even if you have flown through pregnancy and breezed through delivery, you will still need to return progressively to a full exercise programme. The one aspect that does dictate how rapidly you will return to full exercise is how fit you were *before* conception and how dedicated you were to maintaining your conditioning *during* pregnancy. All the effort you put in will now pay off as you return to full fitness much more rapidly than if you had done nothing for the past nine months, or more.

The exertions of childbirth combined with the dramatic changes in your hormones and the challenges of looking after a new baby may leave you very fatigued. As such, there is no one-size-fits-all when it comes to a post-partum exercise programme. Altering your programme to allow for those days when you really don't feel up for it, and those days you do, will ensure you optimize your physical and emotional well-being. As always, that doesn't mean 'do nothing'! You should remain as active as possible every day – even if it means just taking a brisk walk for 30 minutes or so – in order to help accelerate your recovery. Think of your exercise programme as a meal that you can eat in a single sitting or divide into snacks that you can consume across the day. You will gain similar benefits by arranging your exercise into more manageable packages.

Variety remains the spice of life, and making your workouts much easier to consume can be a major motivating factor. So, for example, use interval and fartlek (see page 33) to add spice to your aerobic workouts, and don't stick to the same exercise if it's getting a bit tedious. One of the best ways to add variety and enjoyment to your workout is to join a class and there is a growing number of mother and baby classes that create a fabulous opportunity for you and your baby to bond and exercise together. One of the most important benefits of classes is the social interaction and sharing of a common purpose and experience, which can significantly enhance your quality of life, as you may feel isolated and alone during the post-partum period.

Remember, exercise is crucial for your physical, mental and emotional health and well-being, as well as helping with social integration. The more active you can be during the post-partum period, the faster you will recover, the better and happier you will feel, the easier you will be able to cope with your new responsibilities, and, most importantly, the more you will enjoy being a new mum.

EXERCISE IN WEEKS 1 TO 3 OF THE POST-PARTUM PERIOD

Aerobic:	30 minutes at least 5 days per week. Progress slowly, starting with slow walking and gradually increase the duration of your walks. Divide the 30 minutes into smaller packages.
Abdominal and back strength:	3 times daily
Pelvic floor:	3 to 4 times daily

Listen carefully to your body and manage your exercise accordingly. If it feels like it is too much, reduce the duration and/or the intensity. If you feel you can add more exercise, do it slowly and monitor how you cope to make sure you do not overdo it.

EXERCISE IN WEEKS 4 TO 6 (AND BEYOND) OF THE POST-PARTUM PERIOD

Aerobic:	30 minutes at least 5 days per week. Progress slowly, dividing the 30 minutes into smaller packages and using fartlek or interval training when needed.
Strength:	1 to 2 30-minute sessions per week. Progress slowly and consider shorter sessions spread over the day.
Core strength and stability:	2 to 3 sessions per week
Pelvic floor:	3 to 4 times daily

Post-partum FAQs

How will I know if I'm overdoing it?

It is natural to feel fatigued for some time following childbirth. As you move through the post-partum period, you will know what general pregnancy-related fatigue feels like. In contrast, if in response to exercise you feel exhausted and are struggling to recover the day after your session, you have probably pushed yourself a little too hard. Indeed, if your lochia (post-delivery bleeding and discharge) begins to flow more heavily and/or takes on a darker red colour, it may be a sign to take things a bit easier for a few days. There's no need to stop exercising altogether if you feel up to it, simply reduce the frequency, duration and intensity of your programme. As always, listen to your body, and if you begin to feel run-down, don't be afraid to ease back on your exercise to give yourself time to recover.

Will exercise affect my milk production?

Research shows that milk production is unaffected by exercise, even high-intensity exercise. It is important, however, that you maintain a healthy, balanced diet during the post-partum period, and beyond. Cutting down excessively on your calorie intake to return your body to its pre-pregnancy shape and look can reduce your milk production and increase toxins in your milk. The message of the day is this: exercise and a healthy diet is the best way to support you and your baby.

When can I start swimming after childbirth?

Swimming is a fabulous exercise during the post-partum period. However, there are a number of limitations to returning to swimming at this time. If you have tears or wounds from an episiotomy or C-section, you will have to wait until your wound has fully healed. The use of tampons post-partum is not recommended and therefore you may wish to wait until your flow of lochia becomes light or absent. After your first postnatal check (usually six weeks after delivery) is probably a good point at which to return to swimming. As with many aspects of the post-partum period, how quickly you return to swimming will be determined on an individual basis and will depend on your level of fitness pre- and during pregnancy.

How long will it take to get back to the shape I was in before pregnancy?

The answer to this question is related to your level of activity during pregnancy and how active you can be in this post-partum period. For example, how much weight did you gain during pregnancy? The more weight you gained, the longer it will take you to sensibly regain your former shape. What you achieve following the arrival of your baby is related to how much exercise you can do and how well you are able to control your diet with healthy, balanced meals. Every new mum is different and how quickly they return to their pre-pregnancy state will be a very individual journey. Irrespective of your individual response, it is clear that your exercise and diet programme during and post-pregnancy will be key to the speed at which you get back into shape. That said, you should be careful not to push too hard on this return journey or you may put your health at risk. As always, listen to your body.

When should I start running again after delivery?

There is no definitive timeline for when you can begin running after childbirth. In addition to your mode of delivery (vaginal or C-section) and other complications that you may have experienced during delivery (for example an episiotomy), your physical condition and running experience prior to and during pregnancy is important in your return to running. In addition, the better your physical condition prior to delivery, the faster you are likely to be able to return to running. A progressive re-introduction to running is the best way to ensure your return is a safe one. Having established a good walking programme and worked hard on your strength, core strength and stability, and pelvic floor strength, I suggest a transition to either deep-water running and/or trampette bouncing (using bungee bands rather than metal springs provides a gentler return to bouncing). Once you are confident that you have regained your strength and control you can then return to easy running. Again, I suggest a progressive return to running including running on soft, flat surfaces, and the use of an interval or fartlek structure. Do not rush to return; progress slowly and you'll be entering your first running event before you know it!

Can exercise help with the baby blues/postnatal depression after having my baby?

Postnatal depression is a clinical condition that is suffered by some mothers after giving birth. If you are at all concerned, you should always talk with your health professionals (doctor, midwife, health visitor), who can offer support and guidance.

The baby blues (feeling low, alone, isolated, afraid, anxious, etc.) is a term often used for the more common, short-term low mood experienced by new mums in this post-partum period. It can impact on the quality of life for mum, baby and the rest of the family, so it is important to address any concerns you have immediately by talking to your healthcare professionals, family and friends. A little understanding and empathy goes a long way during what can seem like hectic and sometimes challenging times.

Exercise is a wonderful way to reduce the impact of the baby blues and is a very effective treatment for depression and anxiety, as it changes brain chemicals, for example encouraging the release of the 'feel-good' hormones, endorphins. There are lots of other reasons why exercise is a good thing for new mothers, including psychological, physical and social factors, such as:

- improving self-worth and self-confidence.
- exercise classes provide an opportunity to chat with other new mothers, share experiences and have fun.
- improved fitness makes everyday tasks much easier and can improve sleep quality.

Overall, exercise is a wholly positive experience for the new mother and her baby. My recommendation is to join a class and get involved even before birth, so that you have an easy transition afterwards. Check out what antenatal classes are available in your local area, online or via your healthcare team.

PREGNANCY TRIVIA

Hair today, gone tomorrow!

On average, women lose 100 hairs per day; however, during pregnancy a rise in certain hormones leads to a reduction in hair loss. The increased density of hair is short-lived though, as following delivery you will lose hair more rapidly until you are back to your pre-pregnancy bouffant!

In the swim

The old wives' tale that you cannot take your baby swimming until they have had their full course of vaccinations dates back to the days when polio was common and it was believed that busy places, such as swimming pools, led to an increased risk of infection.

The fastest weight-loss programme known to woman!

The delivery of your new bundle of joy results in an instantaneous loss of around 6kg, made up of your baby, placenta and amniotic fluid. Add to this the reduction in the weight of your uterus of 1kg, and the excess fluid you have been carrying during pregnancy, *et voilà* – lightning-speed weight loss!

Post-partum thyroiditis (PPT)

Immediately following the birth, your thyroid hormone levels change. For around 7 to 9 per cent of women, inflammation of the thyroid gland may result in PPT, where the thyroid initially overproduces then begins to underproduce hormones. There are a range of symptoms that can mimic those observed by all new mums, including fatigue and irritability, making early diagnosis difficult. In contrast to the normal post-partum symptoms, PPT can last for several weeks to several months, with normal thyroid function returning within 12 to 18 months. If you are at all worried or concerned about excessive fatigue in the weeks and months following delivery, speak with your healthcare team.

Happy days

Exercise is associated with decreased postnatal depression. However, this is only true if your exercise routine is stress relieving and not stress inducing. Make your activity fun and enjoyable. Make it part of your life as a new mum!

7

Nutrition and Pregnancy

'We are what we eat', but we are also what our parents and grand-parents ate! Recent studies have shown that nutrition during pregnancy appears to be of great importance not just for the impending offspring but, due to genetic programming, for each successive generation to come. It is important, therefore, to make each mouthful you eat count towards your baby's healthy development from pre-conception to birth and beyond.

Fertility and pre-conception care

Infertility

As we have seen in Chapter 1, there are many lifestyle factors that may contribute to difficulties with conception, such as consumption of alcohol and caffeine, smoking, issues with weight and so on. Here we will look more closely at the effects that stress can have on our attempts to conceive, as well as factors such as toxicity and micronutrient deficiency. If you are having problems conceiving, it would be wise to be tested for heavy-metal toxicity, especially lead and cadmium. If you find you have high levels, then get expert advice on detoxification methods from a nutritional therapist or ecological medical practitioner. Micronutrient levels should also be tested. The minerals zinc and selenium are particularly important for fertility, along with vitamin A, B vitamins, vitamin C, vitamin E and essential fatty acids. There are nutritional therapists who specialize in fertility and pre-conception care and it is often found that adjusting a couple's diet and supplementing with certain nutrients can lead to a great many pregnancy success stories.

Whilst diet plays a major role in fertility levels, elevated stress levels are certainly a contributory factor to infertility. When we are stressed, we produce the hormone cortisol. This is made from the hormone pregnenolone, a hormone that is also required to make the hormones oestrogen, progesterone and testosterone. When pregnenolone is preferentially used for cortisol production during high levels of stress, the production of our sex hormones is reduced. Therefore, you should try to reduce your stress levels, along with factors that cause physiological stress of the body's systems, such as smoking, caffeine, alcohol, recreational/illicit drugs and exposure to excessive levels of pesticides and other environmental toxins.

Pre-conception care

There is much we can do to prepare the body for pregnancy in terms of diet and lifestyle changes, and this applies to men as well as women. Sperm takes three months to mature, making those intervening months a critical time to ensure their optimal health. For a woman, her eggs have been in place since before she was born and their health at this point has more to do with the nourishment she received from her mother. However, environmental exposures in the months preceding conception affect how eggs are selected and grow. The periods of egg and sperm maturation and conception are thought to be the most critical points for the health of a foetus.

Of course, many women have unplanned pregnancies and are not aware of the situation until a few weeks after conception. There may well have been consumption of too much alcohol or other risky behaviour but most women will still go on to give birth to healthy normal-weight babies, so don't get too anxious if this is the case for you! However, it is prudent to say that if a woman is intending to get pregnant, there are diet and lifestyle guidelines that it would be wise to follow.

Weight management

As we have already established, achieving a healthy body weight prior to pregnancy is recommended, as being overweight, obese or underweight is associated with an increased risk of numerous complications and may reduce the likelihood of conception.

Dieting during pregnancy is not advisable, as it can lead to a deficiency in nutrients and compromise your baby's growth; it may also lead to increased feelings of exhaustion on the mother's part. Being significantly overweight or obese during pregnancy may lead to complications such as gestational diabetes, hypertension and pre-eclampsia, and there may be added complications during labour and an increased likelihood of an emergency caesarean delivery.

While we have established that a BMI of between 18.5 and 24.9 is recommended, as well as a body fat mass of between 15 and 35 per cent, another helpful measurement that can be used is waist-to-hip ratio. Waist-to-hip ratio is commonly used as an indicator of healthy body weight and is calculated by measuring your waist at the narrowest point and your hips at the widest point. Divide the waist measurement by the hip measurement. A result above 0.85 is considered too high and it is advisable to increase the amount of exercise you do and take a look at your diet.

Nutritional status

When planning your pregnancy, it is advisable to take an in-depth look at your diet, as a good nutritional status at the point of conception is an important determinant of foetal health. No special diet is needed, but the correct balance of macronutrients (protein, fat and carbohydrate) and a plentiful supply of micronutrients (vitamins and minerals) is essential. Also, it is advisable to supplement your diet with certain nutrients.

Folate should be supplemented by anyone planning a pregnancy and should be continued up to the end of the first trimester (12 weeks). A deficiency can lead to developmental problems, such as the baby's neural tube being unable to close properly, causing brain and spinal-cord defects such as spina bifida. So if there is only one change you make to your diet, folate supplementation must be it.

There has, however, been a lot of debate over the best form of supplementation in terms of folic acid or folate. Folic acid is the synthetic form found in supplements and was thought to be the one most easily absorbed by the gut. However, folic acid is not necessarily all converted to the active form by the body and can lead to a substantial amount of unmetabolized folic acid build-up in the bloodstream, which may be detrimental to health. Folate is the naturally occurring form found in food, the majority of which is converted and absorbed in the gut in the form of 5-methyltetrahydrofolate (5-MTHF), so 5-MTHF is now considered the best supplement form and can generally be found under the name methylfolate.

Environmental toxins

Environmental toxins have become an increasing problem and being aware of them and avoiding them where possible is sensible.

- Eat as organically as possible to reduce pesticide intake.
- Wash fruit and vegetables well.
- Avoid swordfish and shark. Other oily fish (salmon, mackerel, sardines, tuna, herring, trout, anchovies) are healthy to eat but should not be consumed more than twice a week due to the possible high levels of mercury, dioxins and PCBs. It is best to

eat the smaller varieties of these fish, as they are less contaminated. Tinned tuna does not count as an oily fish and also contains higher than average levels of mercury. But if you are particularly fond of tinned tuna, guidelines say you can eat up to four medium-sized tins safely per week.

- Avoid packaged or processed meals and foods to reduce exposure to toxins in the packaging and food additives.
- Avoid the use of plastic containers for water and food. Use only BPA-free bottles and containers.
- Only use oils from glass containers.
- Avoid alcohol.
- Do not smoke and avoid secondhand smoke.
- Do not take recreational/illicit drugs.
- Avoid taking medication, especially in the first trimester, but do not stop prescribed medication without first discussing it with your doctor.
- Avoid industrial chemicals from paint fumes, fabrics, furniture and cars. If you buy new furniture (especially beds) and carpeting, air the room well. Consider having air-purifying plants around the house.
- Use toiletries and cosmetics that are paraben and phthalate free.
- Avoid eating too much rice, which can contain high levels of arsenic.
- Consider a filter for tap water.

Nutrition during pregnancy

It may seem a cruel injustice of nature that just when you want to start nurturing your baby with good nutrition you are more than likely feeling nauseous at the thought of eating. What's more, you may well be craving all sorts of things which are less than healthy for you. They say your body knows what it needs, but does it? Many people seem to crave all manner of unhealthy foods. The very important first trimester can therefore be a challenging time to implement a healthy-eating regime.

Energy requirements increase during pregnancy, particularly as the pregnancy progresses, but it must always be remembered that there really is no need to eat for two! Most dietary advice for pregnant women is the same as for non-pregnant women, with a few exceptions. The placenta provides the developing foetus with all its nutritional needs, therefore dietary intake must also provide sufficient nutrition for the mother and for the storage of nutrients to cope with the rapid development of the foetus in the later stages of pregnancy and for lactation.

Macronutrient requirements during pregnancy

Protein
Protein requirements increase during pregnancy but in general most women in the UK eat more than adequate amounts of protein. The rate that protein is deposited during pregnancy increases with each trimester. It is thought that on average an extra 6g of protein is required by the body daily. If necessary, this can easily be achieved by eating an extra egg or a handful of nuts.

For vegans, an increased intake of protein may be harder to achieve, as animal products are the best source of protein. However, if you are following a vegan diet then beans, lentils, grains, nuts and seeds need to be varied and plentiful to provide all the essential amino acids.

Fat
Healthy fats, such as the essential fatty acids omega-3 and -6, are vital for a healthy pregnancy and foetus from pre-conception and through each trimester. They are termed essential as they cannot be made in the body and so must be obtained through diet. A deficiency may increase the risk of pre-eclampsia and premature birth.

Long chain omega-3 fatty acids (DHA and EPA) are key to healthy cell membrane structure, tissue formation and growth, and so are of particular importance for brain, eye and nervous-system development. They may have beneficial effects on birth weight and the duration of your pregnancy, and appear to protect a newborn baby against eczema. Good sources of omega-3 fatty acids are oily fish, nuts, seeds, green leafy vegetables, avocados, olives and olive oil, and meat and dairy from grass-fed cattle. Do not supplement with cod liver oil, as this contains retinol.

Trans-fats or hydrogenated fats are toxic to the body in high amounts and may well have a negative effect on pregnancy. These manufactured fats can be found in meat products, some margarine, some processed foods, biscuits, cakes, sweets and fried foods, such as doughnuts and French fries. So beware – a large intake of trans-fats can block the uptake of the all-important essential fatty acids.

Carbohydrates

Carbohydrates include sugars and starches and both are broken down to glucose on digestion. Sugars and starches are present in vegetables, fruit and grains. Eating these foods in their whole form will supply numerous nutrients and plenty of fibre. Avoid consuming too many in their refined form, such as concentrated fruit juices and fruit smoothies, products made from white flour (bread, pasta, cakes, biscuits), and refined cereals and rice that have no fibre and very little in the way of nutrient value. Choose wholegrain varieties of bread, pasta, cereals and rice, and eat whole fruit whenever possible.

Constipation can be an issue during pregnancy and should be avoided where possible. Vegetables, fruits and whole grains can be useful for maintaining regular bowel movements, and ground flax-seeds and psyllium husks can also be useful additions to the diet to combat constipation.

IMPORTANT MICRONUTRIENTS DURING PREGNANCY

Nutrient	Top food sources	Functions
Vitamin A (retinol) (beta-carotene – converts to vitamin A)	Eggs, meat, oily fish, dairy, yellow and dark-green leafy vegetables and fruit (carrots, red peppers, spinach, mango, papaya, apricots)	Important for cell growth, skin and membrane development, and metabolic functions. **Take care:** it is stored in the body and the accumulation of too much can lead to birth defects. Avoid liver and liver products that are high in retinol. Do not take supplements containing retinol – only beta-carotene.
Vitamin B$_1$ (thiamine)	Pork, milk, cheese, eggs, wholegrain cereals, brown rice, beans, nuts, barley, lentils, vegetables and fruit, dried fruit	Important in the **third trimester** for the release of energy from the body's cells.
Vitamin B$_2$ (riboflavin)	Milk, eggs, brown rice, mushrooms, green leafy vegetables, meat and fish	Needed throughout pregnancy for energy requirements.
Vitamin B$_6$ (pyridoxine)	Milk, eggs, whole grains, wheatgerm, vegetables – especially cruciferous – meat, yeast, beans, walnuts	Important in the release of energy from food, protein metabolism, formation of haemoglobin, and hormone balance. Can help to ease nausea.

Nutrient	Top food sources	Functions
Vitamin B$_9$ (folate)	Green leafy vegetables, peas, chickpeas, yeast extract, brown rice, bananas, oranges	Important in pre-conception and the **first trimester** for reducing the risk of neural-tube defects such as spina bifida. Supplement with 400mcg daily until the twelfth week.
Vitamin C	Fruit and vegetables, especially sprouted seeds and beans, broccoli, cabbage, potatoes, tomatoes, blackcurrants, oranges, kiwi, red and black berries	Important for tissue growth and repair, collagen production, immunity function, and aids the absorption of non-haem iron. Increase in demand in the **third trimester**. Assists the liver in the detoxification of heavy metals.
Vitamin D	Sunlight, oily fish, eggs	Assists calcium in the formation of strong bones and teeth. Reduces the risk of pre-eclampsia. Important in the **second and third trimesters**. The NHS recommends pregnant women supplement with 10mcg a day.

Nutrient	Top food sources	Functions
Vitamin K	Spinach, cabbage, cauliflower, peas, cereals	Useful in the **third trimester** to help with blood clotting.
Calcium*	Dairy, almonds, sardines with bones, green leafy vegetables, rhubarb, beans, blackstrap molasses	Absorption of calcium increases during pregnancy. Especially important in the **second trimester** for forming baby's bones and teeth. Reduces the risk of pre-eclampsia and pre-term birth.
Iron	Haem-iron – meat, kidneys, heart, poultry and fish Non-haem iron – wheat, beans and lentils, vegetables – especially green leafy vegetables – fruit, dairy	Important in the production of red blood cells used for transporting oxygen to the placenta and foetus. Many pregnant women become anaemic. Ensure iron levels are checked regularly, especially if you become pale and extra tired.
Iodine**	Seaweed, seafood (fish), iodized salt, vegetables and cereals grown in iodine-rich soil	Important for thyroid function and brain development. Important in the **first and second trimesters**.

Nutrient	Top food sources	Functions
Magnesium	Soya, nuts, green leafy vegetables, whole grains, meat, fish, sunflower seeds, figs	Required for bone formation. A deficiency may contribute to pre-eclampsia. Important in the **third trimester** to prepare for breastfeeding.
Copper	Eggs, whole wheat, beans, beetroot, fish, spinach, asparagus, nuts	Important for bone formation. A constituent of breast milk.
Selenium	Brazil nuts, vegetables, chicken, egg yolks, whole grains, milk, mushrooms, pulses, meat, fish	Important in the **first trimester**, as a deficiency may be linked to miscarriage.

* **Calcium** is taken from the bones of the mother to cope with the increased demand during pregnancy. This deficit will later be replenished but teenage girls who become pregnant need supplementation of calcium, as their bones have not yet calcified sufficiently to meet the demands of pregnancy and this may cause them to have bone-density problems in later years.

** **Iodine** is depleted in much of the soil around the world. Recent research suggests that around 67 per cent of the UK's pregnant women are iodine deficient. This can have implications for the foetus's brain development and cognitive skills later in childhood. At present, iodine supplementation is not recommended as a matter of course but the consumption of iodine-rich foods (see table) is recommended, especially seaweed. Do not supplement with kelp, as levels of iodine can vary, with some sources delivering excessive amounts.

Blood sugar control

Uncontrolled blood-glucose levels during pregnancy can increase the risk of gestational diabetes, which can cause complications during delivery and may increase the risk of the child developing type-2 diabetes later in life.

Eat a low-glycaemic diet – choose the foods recommended in the carbohydrate information on page 177 (wholefood and -grain varieties), which release sugars slowly into the bloodstream in a controlled manner. Eat healthy fats and protein alongside carbohydrates to slow down digestion time. If you do choose to eat something sugary (a high glycaemic food), it is best to eat it immediately after a meal.

Try to avoid energy drinks, other sugary drinks or diet fizzy drinks.

Caffeine

In recent years, caffeine has increasingly been the subject of research in many pregnancy studies. There is still insufficient evidence to make conclusive recommendations but as any caffeine consumed passes freely to the baby it would be wise to follow current advice. Research has shown that there may be a link between high caffeine intake and low-birth-weight babies. One piece of research has even suggested that consumption of three caffeinated drinks daily by both parents prior to conception may increase the risk of early miscarriage. Guidelines for pregnant women are for no more than 200mg of caffeine per day (approximately 2 mugs tea/coffee) but in the light of recent research it may be advisable to limit this further. Remember that energy drinks, some soft drinks and green tea contain caffeine too. Check food packaging labels!

Alcohol

If you are planning to become pregnant or are pregnant, then you should refrain from drinking any alcohol. Alcohol consumption can lead to long-term harm to the baby, with the risk increasing the more you drink.

Peanuts

Unless you have an allergy to these, there is no reason to avoid them. The causes of nut allergies in children are still not clearly understood but it is now agreed that if nuts are avoided during pregnancy, it may increase the risk of your baby developing an allergy.

Morning sickness

As so many pregnant women complain – if only it were just in the morning! Nausea and sickness can be miserable but some dietary tricks can help to control the problem to some extent.

- Try to eat little and often, as this will help to balance your blood sugar, which can keep nausea at bay. Don't worry too much if your diet is less than balanced – your baby will gain its nutrition from your stores of nutrients.
- Try to ensure that you don't give in to cravings for processed, unhealthy foods. We often crave carbohydrate foods, but aim to eat these in their healthier state, for example wholegrain bread, jacket potatoes, fresh fruit and vegetables.
- Making juices or smoothies can often be a palatable way of gaining nutrients when appetite is impaired.
- Ginger has been shown to alleviate nausea and sickness, as it calms the digestive tract and aids blood-sugar control. Adding fresh or dried ginger to food may be a good way of consuming it. You can also make a ginger tea by infusing a couple of slices of ginger root in hot water and sipping it throughout the day.

Microbiota

The microbiome is the term for the collection of microbiota (bacteria) that reside within the human body. It has been the subject of many studies in recent years and it is certainly clear that beneficial microbiota play a significant role in human health by aiding digestion, stimulating the immune system and protecting the gut from pathogens. There has been growing interest in the influence of a mother's microbiome on the newborn. It appears that the balance of a mother's microbiota and their interaction within her body before conception, during gestation and immediately before and after birth have profound effects on the developing immune system. It is thought that this is related to the theory of 'foetal programming', whereby at critical points in early development genes are expressed (switched on) in response to environmental conditions.

Babies who are born vaginally are mainly exposed to microbiota that originate from their mother and these will begin the generally healthy colonization of the baby's gut, which until now had been sterile. Those delivered by caesarean acquire their microbiota mainly from their environment. It is now considered wise to inoculate your newborn baby orally with beneficial probiotics if born by caesarean. Probiotics are microbiota similar to those found in the human body, which are believed to exert health benefits when consumed. Every person has a unique microbiome that was influenced initially by the microbiota we were introduced to at birth and in our early years.

Research has investigated the safety of supplementing probiotics during pregnancy, in regard to premature birth, the colonization of the newborn gut and the long-term effects on the child's health. It appears to be safe for pregnant women to supplement with probiotics. Oral administration of *Lactobacillus rhamnosus* (strain LGG) to mothers during pregnancy was found in one study to temporarily colonize the gut of newborn babies for up to 24 months, which may provide protection from some infections. Another study found that women taking probiotics during pregnancy had a significantly reduced risk of gestational diabetes. Long term it is thought that this may offer protection from health consequences as diverse as eczema, allergic rhinitis and inflammatory bowel disease, but this research is ongoing.

Perhaps the easiest and safest way of helping to create a healthy microbiome is to consume pre- and probiotic foods. Prebiotic foods promote the growth of our beneficial microbiota and are those containing soluble fibres such as Jerusalem artichokes, leeks, onions, beans, peas, lentils and oats. Probiotic foods are fermented and include live yogurt, kefir, kombucha, sauerkraut, miso and kimchi. These help to colonize our gut with beneficial microbiota.

The recipes in the following chapter have been designed to include an array of nutrients that are beneficial during pregnancy. We have highlighted with each recipe the particular helpful effects of these nutrients, including, in some cases, the trimester when the nutrient is of most importance. Each recipe is simple, easy to follow and does not require any difficult-to-find ingredients.

8

Bump It Up Recipes

Start the day well

Munch a good lunch

Super suppers

Bump It Up staples

Nausea settlers

Good foods to include in your diet   218
Foods to avoid   220

Start the day well

Red berry, lemon and chia-seed smoothie

serves 2

takes 15 minutes

Fantastically high in phytonutrients, protein and healthy fats, this smoothie ticks all the boxes for a delicious, nutritious, refreshing start to your day. Water makes a lighter-tasting drink and is all too frequently overlooked in smoothies. So if you are not so keen on milk, try this variation.

100g strawberries, hulled
100g raspberries
100g blueberries
juice of ½ a lemon
approx. 500ml water
2 tbs ground almonds
1 tbs chia seeds

Place the hulled strawberries, raspberries and blueberries in a Nutribullet or blender, add the lemon juice, water, almonds and chia seeds, and blend until smooth.

Spinach, lentil and flaked-salmon omelette

serves 2

takes 15 minutes

A tasty brunch-style breakfast that is a good start to a healthy-eating day. Spinach will supply you with some iron and the vitamin C in the pepper will enhance its absorption. Eggs and salmon will give a boost to that all-important protein intake, while the salmon also delivers some healthy omega-3 fatty acids.

The lentils in this recipe will add some essential fibre to your diet, which is great for getting a sluggish gut moving. It's useful to have some cooked lentils in your fridge, as they are great to use in salads; added to soups, casseroles or omelettes, they add protein and fibre. Alternatively, try using tinned lentils.

4 free-range eggs
2 tbs milk
sea salt and freshly ground black pepper
a little olive oil
80g cooked lentils
½ red pepper, sliced
50g spinach
100g flaked cooked salmon

Break the eggs into a jug, whisk well with the milk and seasoning. In a small pan, heat a little olive oil, add the lentils and red peppers and cook for 5 minutes over a medium heat.

Heat a little more olive oil in a medium non-stick pan and when hot pour in the egg mix to make the omelette. Gently pull the set egg mix in to allow the liquid egg to fill the exposed areas.

It will only take a matter of minutes for the egg to set and when it has, spoon the warmed lentil mix across the top of the omelette and add the spinach leaves and the flaked salmon. Fold the cooked omelette over and serve cut in half, making one large wedge per person.

Home-made nut and seed muesli

makes 850g

takes 15 minutes

You will definitely feel virtuous after eating this muesli for break-fast. Packed with grains, nuts and seeds, you'll be gaining plenty of B vitamins, minerals and essential fatty acids. Cinnamon adds a touch of sweetness, along with the dried fruit, so there will be no need for any added sugar. If you want a totally gluten-free muesli, remove the rye and increase the quantity of rolled gluten-free oats.

200g rolled oats

100g rye flakes

50g quinoa flakes

50g hemp seeds

50g pumpkin seeds

50g sunflower seeds

150g dried fruits, for example figs, golden raisins, apricots, cherries, pomegranate, mango – the choice is yours

150g nuts, for example almonds, walnuts, macadamias, hazelnuts, brazils, pecans – the choice is yours – roughly chopped

50g coconut flakes

1 tsp ground cinnamon

In a large bowl, mix together all of the above ingredients and then store in an airtight container. Serve with nut, grain or dairy milk; use hot milk in the winter.

To transform this into Bircher muesli, which has a softer texture, place a portion of the mixture in a bowl, grate in an apple and a pear and combine well. Add 4 tbs of Greek yogurt and a little fruit juice or milk. Mix well again and leave in the fridge overnight before enjoy-ing for breakfast the next day.

Coconut, banana and ginger smoothie

serves 2

takes 10 minutes

This is a good smoothie for anyone who is lactose intolerant or vegan. Creamy, with a bit of a tasty zing from the ginger and lime juice, this is a nourishing and filling drink that is packed with natural goodness and rich in good fats and bone–building minerals.

On a hot day, try cutting up and freezing the bananas before making this for a deliciously fresh, chilled drink.

2–3 ripe bananas
5cm fresh ginger, peeled and chopped
juice of 1 lime
400ml tinned coconut milk, chilled

Place the bananas, ginger and lime in a blender or Nutribullet, then add the coconut milk and blitz until smooth and creamy. If the smoothie is too thick, add a little water to adjust.

Sunrise fruit salad with spiced ground-seed sprinkle

serves 2

takes 15 minutes

Pimp your fruit salad with the unusual but delicious addition of ground seeds. This is a veritable fruit-fest, packed with vitamin C and beta-carotene plus many important minerals including folate. Unusually, this fruit salad also has protein from the important addition of the seeds. Papaya also contains an enzyme that aids the digestion of the seeds.

2 fresh apricots, de-stoned (out of season, use dried apricots)
¼ melon, de-seeded, peeled and diced
½ papaya, de-seeded, peeled and diced
½ mango, de-stoned, peeled and diced
1 tsp sesame seeds
1 tsp hemp seeds
1 tsp poppy seeds
½ tsp cinnamon
juice of 1 lime

Prepare and cut the fruit into equal-sized pieces, place in a large bowl and gently mix. Put all the seeds in a Nutribullet or blender and blitz until roughly ground. Sprinkle the mix over the fruits along with the cinnamon and lime juice, then mix and serve.

Munch a good lunch

Miso broth with vegetables and udon noodles

serves 2

takes 30 minutes

This simple recipe is comforting, warming and perfect for days when your body just wants clean fresh flavours that are easy to digest. Do not feel restricted to the vegetables that are listed; add or exchange for other favourites such as chard, asparagus, beans or mangetout – and if you feel a protein boost is needed, add some shredded cooked chicken, sliced ribbons of cooked beef or flaked cooked fish to the broth.

Miso is made from fermented soya beans and is excellent for gut health as it helps to top up beneficial gut microflora. Onions, garlic, cabbage and mushrooms are superfoods that also play an important role in keeping the gut and its abundant microflora healthy. And here's a tip: if you place your mushrooms in sunlight, they will naturally increase their vitamin D content.

5cm fresh ginger, peeled and grated or finely chopped
1 small onion, finely sliced into moons
1 small garlic clove, crushed
1 tbs soy sauce
2 tbs miso paste
100g udon noodles
2 spring onions, trimmed and sliced into thin rings
100g of your favourite mushrooms, sliced if large
50g spinach
50g cabbage, finely sliced
50g peas
1 tbs toasted sesame seeds

In a medium-sized pot, place the ginger, onion, garlic, soy sauce and 750ml water. Mix well, bring to the boil and then simmer for 10 minutes. Once the broth has cooled a little, add the miso paste and stir to dissolve. Don't let the miso boil, as this will destroy the live enzymes. Heat another pan of water and cook the noodles for 6 minutes or according to the packet instructions.

To the miso pot, add the spring onions, mushrooms, spinach, cabbage and peas. Bring to a simmer and then turn the heat off.

When the noodles are cooked, drain, divide between two bowls and ladle on the broth and vegetables. Top with the sesame seeds and serve.

Butter bean, avocado and tomato salad with feta

serves 2

takes 35 minutes

Avocados are a great versatile superfood, a real treasure trove of nutrients, and especially beneficial during early pregnancy due to the folate and healthy fats they contain. They can easily be incorporated into your daily diet. Slice and add to a salad, simply mash the flesh on to hot toast, or make a spicy guacamole dip. This salad is a perfect balance of protein, fats, carbohydrate and colourful vegetables to help keep you energized.

400g tin butter beans, drained and rinsed
200g cherry tomatoes, halved
small bunch flat-leaf parsley, chopped
1 red chilli, finely diced (optional)
1 slice sourdough bread, cut into cubes
juice of 1 lemon
2 tbs olive oil
sea salt and freshly ground black pepper

1 ripe avocado, de-stoned, peeled and sliced
25g/handful of sprouted seed greens or cress
50g feta, cubed

In a bowl, place the butter beans, cherry tomatoes, chopped parsley, optional chilli, cubed sourdough, lemon juice, olive oil and seasoning. Mix well and leave to sit for 30 minutes. This will allow the flavours to blend. When ready to serve, dice the avocado and add to the salad with the sprouted seed greens. Toss and serve with feta on the side.

Mexican refried beans with spinach and poached egg

serves 2

takes 40 minutes

If you visit Mexico, this dish will be served for breakfast, lunch and supper. It is a healthy, economical staple that can usually be cooked from the store cupboard, so stock up for that day when you don't have the time or the inclination to shop.

Nutritionally, this is an excellent meal because by adding beans and lentils to a dish you are providing plenty of fibre, protein and carbohydrates. Fibre binds to any toxins in the gut and this helps to eliminate them from the body before they are absorbed into the bloodstream.

1 tbs olive oil
1 onion, chopped
1 clove garlic, crushed
1 red chilli, finely diced
1 red pepper, chopped
400g tin mixed beans, drained and rinsed, or 125g dried mixed beans, cooked

1 tsp cumin
1 tsp paprika
2 free-range eggs
50g spinach
small bunch coriander, chopped
1 lime, ½ juiced

Heat the olive oil in a large pan and add the chopped onion, garlic, chilli and red pepper. Sweat for 5 minutes until just soft. Roughly break up the beans with the back of a fork or masher and add to the pan along with the spices and mix well. Add 100ml water and cook for 15 minutes, or until the water has evaporated. Set aside.

Bring a medium pan of water to the boil, reduce the heat to low and when the water is completely still (not bubbling) carefully crack an egg, break it in half and lower the egg into the water as closely as possible, which will help to keep the white intact. Place a lid on the pan and leave to poach on a very low heat for 8 minutes for a hard yolk. When cooked, remove the egg with a slotted spoon and rest on kitchen paper to absorb any excess moisture. Do the same with the second egg.

When the eggs are almost ready, add the spinach, chopped coriander and the juice from half the lime to the beans. Fry for a further 2 minutes and serve the beans topped with the poached egg. Add a few coriander sprigs and a wedge of lime to finish.

Pearl barley and green vegetable–style risotto with added chicken shreds (optional)

serves 2

takes 30 minutes

Pearl barley is an often overlooked grain. It works very well as a replacement for Arborio rice and adds texture and a light nutty flavour. A top tip: do not use polished pearl barley as it has had its husk removed and it's the husk that adds natural extra roughage to your diet. There is a concern that some rice has high arsenic levels, so pearl barley is a safe grain to use. And remember, the quality of your stock will make all the difference to the taste and nutritional benefits of your food, so turn to page 207 for our recipe.

1 tbs olive oil
1 onion, finely diced
1 clove garlic, crushed
150g pearl barley
600ml chicken or vegetable stock
200g cooked chicken, shredded (optional)
1 leek, finely sliced
75g green cabbage, finely sliced
75g broccoli florets
75g peas
sea salt and freshly ground pepper
ground seaweed
75g Parmesan cheese

Heat the olive oil in a medium saucepan and add the onion and garlic. Cook for 5 minutes until soft. Add the pearl barley, mix well, then pour in the chicken or vegetable stock and bring to a simmer. Cook for 12 minutes, stirring occasionally to ensure even cooking. Test the pearl barley; it should be almost soft.

Next, if using shredded chicken, mix it in well and cook for a further 2 minutes. Add the leek, cabbage, broccoli and peas, mix well and simmer for a further 3 minutes for al dente vegetables, or 6 minutes for soft vegetables. Season with salt, pepper and seaweed. Just before serving, stir in half the Parmesan and serve the remainder sprinkled on top.

Bruschetta topped with tinned sardines, tomato and avocado, with a watercress and lemon dressing

serves 2

takes 20 minutes

Tinned sardines usually contain the bones of the fish, which are incredibly soft, edible and a good source of calcium. Watercress is a wonderful green leafy vegetable that contains very good levels of vitamins A and C, along with excellent levels of vitamin K, which is important for bone and brain health. Serve this as a snack or as a super-boosting healthy starter at a gathering.

2 handfuls of watercress
juice of 1 lemon
2 tbs olive oil
1 tsp sesame seeds
1 tbs Greek yogurt
sea salt and freshly ground pepper
2 slices toasted sourdough bread
2 tomatoes, sliced
1 avocado, de-stoned, peeled and sliced
200g tin sardines (in brine)

In a small blender, or with a hand-held blender, blitz together half the watercress with the lemon juice, olive oil, sesame seeds, Greek yogurt and seasoning until fully blended. On the hot toasted sourdough, brush a little of the dressing and then add the sliced tomato, avocado and sardines. Add the remaining watercress and drizzle the rest of the dressing on top.

Super suppers

Rump steak ribbons with coconut rice and vegetable stir-fry

serves 2

takes 25–40 minutes

Whenever you have a classic steak for supper, cook twice the amount and then just reserve half to cut into ribbons for this hot tasty meal. Any steak can be used; we just favour rump for its flavour. Red meat is the best way to top up iron levels but eat in moderation. Stir-fried vegetables are quick and easy, and this speedy way of cooking also retains more of the nutrients in the food.

½ tin coconut milk, mixed with 100ml of water
150g brown or white basmati rice
1 tbs olive oil
1 clove garlic, crushed
1 red chilli, finely diced
5cm ginger, peeled and grated or finely chopped
150g rump steak, cooked and cut into thin ribbons/strips
½ red pepper, sliced into thin strips
50g broccoli, chopped into small florets
50g cabbage, shredded
50g beansprouts
small bunch coriander, chopped
1 lime, cut in half

Pour the coconut milk and 100ml of water into a pan, add the rice and bring to a simmer. Stir so that all the hard coconut milk has melted. (You will need to simmer for 25–30 minutes for brown rice or 10 minutes for white rice, stirring occasionally.) Then place a lid on the pan and allow to sit for 5 minutes. The rice should then be perfectly cooked and all the coconut liquid absorbed.

In a wok, heat the oil, add the garlic, chilli and ginger and cook for 2 minutes. Then add the beef strips and red pepper. Toss well and cook on a high heat for 2 minutes. Finally, add the broccoli, cabbage and beansprouts. Keep the heat high, toss frequently and cook for another 2 minutes. Finally, add the coriander and serve with the coconut rice and lime.

Ginger chicken soba noodles with bok choi and peas

serves 2

takes 25 minutes

Buy good-quality chicken – it is worth spending that bit more on high-welfare meat and cutting down on your portion size to budget for this. Quality chicken broth will add depth of flavour and many nutrients to this dish; ginger also adds a variety of health benefits, making this a tasty bowl of rainbow goodness. Buckwheat noodles are delicious and contain the mineral manganese, which helps form bone and cartilage.

drizzle of olive oil
2 chicken breasts, skin on
800ml chicken broth
100g buckwheat soba noodles
5cm ginger, peeled and finely cut into matchsticks
1 clove garlic, crushed
75g small mushrooms
2 heads of bok choi, cut into quarters
50g peas
2 handfuls of beansprouts
1 red chilli, finely diced

small bunch coriander, chopped
2 spring onions, sliced
1 tsp toasted sesame seeds
sea salt, freshly ground pepper and ground seaweed

Heat the drizzle of oil in a non-stick pan, place the chicken breasts skin side down in the pan and sear for 3 minutes. Then reduce the heat and cook for a further 6 minutes (the skin should be golden and crunchy). Turn and cook on the other side for 5 minutes before removing from the heat.

Pour the chicken broth into two separate pans and bring to a simmer. Add the noodles to one pan and cook according to the packet instructions.

In the other broth pot, add the ginger, garlic, mushrooms, bok choi and peas and simmer for 2 minutes.

Drain the noodle cooking broth into the vegetable cooking broth pan and divide the noodles between two large bowls. Then drain the vegetable broth back into the empty pan and share the vegetables between the two bowls. Bring the broth back to the boil. Slice the cooked chicken breast and lay it on top of the vegetables. Finally, ladle in the stock to just below the vegetables. Top with the beansprouts, diced chilli, coriander, spring onions and a sprinkling of sesame seeds, and season with the salt, pepper and seaweed.

Salmon cakes with chia seeds, broccoli and cashew–nut stir-fry

serves 2

takes 20 minutes

These easy-to-prepare salmon cakes contain an abundance of healthy fats. Salmon and chia seeds are both high in omega-3, which will contribute to your baby's brain development. As chia seeds have no real flavour, try using them in your everyday cooking, as they are so nutritious and can help to thicken soups, casseroles and stewed fruits.

Turmeric is a spice known for its amazing health benefits, including its anti-inflammatory properties. So if you have aching joints, using turmeric in your cooking may help.

250g skinless salmon
½ tsp ground turmeric, or 2.5cm grated if fresh
sea salt and freshly ground black pepper
½ tbs chia seeds
½ tbs sesame seeds
½ tbs coconut oil
100g broccoli florets
50g chopped cashew nuts
1 tsp sesame oil

Place the salmon, turmeric and seasoning in a food processor and pulse until roughly chopped. Transfer to a mixing bowl; add the chia and sesame seeds (they are best mixed together using your hands for an even blend). Divide the mixture in two and shape into patties about 3cm thick.

Heat the coconut oil in a large non-stick pan, add the salmon cakes and cook for 4 minutes on each side. Then add the broccoli florets and cook together with the fishcakes for another 5 minutes or until they are golden. Remove the salmon cakes when cooked, then add the cashew nuts and sesame oil to the pan, toss to heat through and serve with the salmon cakes.

Hot tuna butternut Niçoise

serves 2

takes 30 minutes

Enjoy this colourful Mediterranean-inspired meal served hot or warm. It is super-quick and simple to prepare. Tuna is an oily fish that is healthy when eaten in moderation. It can be high in mercury, so it is advisable to consume tuna less often than smaller oily fish.

200g butternut squash, peeled
3 tbs olive oil
2 sprigs thyme, leaves picked off twig
sea salt and freshly ground black pepper
2 x 125g fresh tuna steak (tinned can be an option but it makes a totally different-tasting dish)
2 tomatoes, cut into quarters
small bunch parsley, chopped
1 baby gem, cut into wedges
black olives
3 tbs balsamic vinegar
1 lemon, cut into wedges

Preheat the oven to 200°C, gas mark 7, chop the butternut squash into slim wedges and place in a roasting pan with 1 tbs olive oil and the thyme and seasoning. Toss well to coat and roast in the oven for 20 minutes, or until soft.

Sear the tuna steaks on each side in a hot non-stick pan for 5 minutes for well done. On a large platter, arrange the cooked butternut squash, prepared tomatoes, parsley, baby gem, olives, seasoning and pour the remaining olive oil and balsamic vinegar over. Top with the tuna steaks and lemon wedges.

Moroccan lamb with apricots, minted almond couscous and watermelon

serves 4

takes 2 hours

When you feel like entertaining, this is an easy dish to prepare. It can be cooked in advance and then reheated and finished off just before serving. The lamb freezes well if you want to do some batch cooking.

Moroccan food is full of healthy spices and the inclusion of ground seeds to thicken the dish adds even more protein to this meal. Both the apricot and watermelon are high in phytonutrients and the watermelon contains lycopene, which is important for cardiovascular and bone health. Another component of watermelon, citrulline, converts to the amino acid arginine, which improves blood flow, an important consideration in pregnancy.

1 tbs olive oil

500g lean braising lamb, cut into chunks

1 clove garlic, crushed

1 onion, diced

1 red chilli, finely diced

5cm ginger, peeled and finely diced

1 tsp ground cumin

1 tsp ground coriander

1 tsp cinnamon

2 tbs ground-seed sprinkle (see page 212)

100g dried apricots

sea salt and freshly ground black pepper

750ml lamb or vegetable stock

400g couscous

20g toasted flaked almonds

small bunch mint, chopped

2 slices watermelon, cut into cubes

Preheat the oven to 170°C, gas mark 5. Heat the olive oil in an oven-proof pan on the hob, add the lamb and cook on a high heat until browned. Reduce the heat to medium-low, add the garlic, onion and chilli and cook for a further 5 minutes, or until the onions are soft. Add the ginger, cumin, coriander, cinnamon and ground-seed sprinkle and mix well. Then add the apricots and seasoning and pour in the stock until the meat is just covered. Mix well again, place a lid on and cook in the oven for 1½ hours, or until the meat is tender.

Place the couscous in a bowl and just cover with boiling water, stir well, cover and keep warm for 10 minutes. When ready, transfer the couscous to a large, warm, open bowl, make a well in the centre and ladle in the Moroccan lamb. Top with the almonds and chopped mint and place the cubed watermelon around the edge. Serve at the table, allowing everyone to help themselves.

Bump It Up staples

Super broths and Asian-style quick soups

makes approximately 1 litre

4–12 hours

Super broths have become very popular because they can be converted into Asian-style quick soups and served in meal-sized Buddha bowls very easily. They are light, refreshing and nourishing and have no end of health benefits. In particular, these broths can improve gut health and may even improve skin elasticity – perhaps helping to keep those stretch marks at bay!

The cider vinegar or lemon juice used in the recipe helps to extract the all-important minerals from the bones used. Make a batch of your chosen broth and then freeze into 500ml portions so that you always have a quantity of good home-made broth to use in all your cooking.

When serving as a soup, you can vary the tastes and flavours by adding different vegetables and spices to the broth (such as chillies, for a little heat).

2kg bones – beef, chicken, turkey, lamb, pork or fish – *never* **mix bones**

2 onions, chopped

2 carrots, chopped

handful of celery tops

1–2 cloves garlic, whole

1 bouquet garni: a parsley stalk, bay leaf, marjoram and thyme tied together in a bundle

sea salt

1 tsp peppercorns

1 tbs cider vinegar or juice of ½ a lemon

If you want a brown broth, use beef, lamb or pork. Preheat the oven to 200°C, gas mark 7, place the bones in a roasting tray and roast for 1 hour, turning to ensure even browning all over, then follow the recipe below for the paler broth.

For a paler-looking, lighter-flavoured broth, place the chicken, turkey or fish bones in a large stockpot; add the roughly chopped vegetables, bouquet garni and seasoning, then cover with water; add the vinegar or lemon juice and bring to the boil. Remove and discard any scum that may float to the surface. Reduce the heat, cover with a lid and simmer for between 4 and 12 hours – the longer the better, so the more nutritious and flavoursome your broth will be. If you have an Aga, putting this in the low oven overnight works a treat.

When cooked, strain the broth through a fine strainer, or colander with a piece of muslin. Use immediately, or cool and place in the fridge, where it can be stored for several days. Alternatively, you can freeze the broth. Usually, once cool, a layer of fat will settle on top, which is good as it stops air getting to the broth. Just lift off the hard-set fat before using.

Four-seed spelt soda bread

serves 2

takes 1 hour

Healthy bread is hard to find in the shops. If you make your own, you know exactly what the ingredients are – and there are no hidden stabilizers or sugars in this bread! It is simple to make and full of healthy seeds for added omega-3 fatty acids.

250ml milk
1 tsp lemon juice
300g spelt flour
25g sunflower seeds, ground
25g pumpkin seeds, ground
25g sesame seeds, ground
25g hemp seeds, ground
pinch of salt
2 tsp bicarbonate of soda

Preheat the oven to 200°C, gas mark 7. Add the milk to the lemon juice and leave to react and split. This will take about 10 minutes. Meanwhile, place the spelt, ground seeds, salt and bicarbonate of soda in a large bowl and mix until evenly blended. Add the milk mixture and, by hand, combine together.

Lightly dust the work surface with flour and knead the dough for about 3 minutes, or until you have an even texture. Shape the dough into a ball and place on to a lightly floured baking sheet. Cut a cross on the top with a sharp knife, then place in the middle of the oven and bake for 20 minutes. Then reduce the oven to 180°C, gas mark 6, and cook for a further 20 minutes. To check if the bread is cooked, tap the base and it should sound hollow. If it doesn't, return to the oven for a little longer.

Fruitjacks

serves 2–4

takes 30 minutes

A treat for when you crave some sweetness. The chopped dates add a natural, sweet flavour that sometimes our bodies hanker after. These really are much better for you than a shop-bought biscuit, cake or cereal bar, as the sugar content is lower and there are no hidden ingredients.

100g butter
50g brown sugar
2 tbs golden syrup
150g oats
200g dried dates, or other favourite dried fruits, chopped

Preheat the oven to 170°C, gas mark 5. Line a small baking sheet with parchment. In a saucepan, place the butter, sugar and golden syrup and gently heat until melted and blended together. Add the oats and chopped dried fruits and mix well, coating everything in the syrup mixture.

Transfer to the baking sheet and spread out until roughly even. Place in the oven and bake for 20 minutes, or until golden. Remove and allow to cool a little before carefully cutting into approximately 8 pieces. Leave to cool completely before lifting out and cutting into smaller pieces. Store in an airtight container for up to 5 days.

Fresh fruit and chia–seed sugarless jam

makes a large jar

takes 20 minutes

Enjoy this delicious jam that has no added sugars. What's more, you even have the benefits of some ultra-healthy chia seeds. If you have a really sweet tooth, it may take you a while to fully appreciate it, but try weaning yourself off sugar, as it is very damaging.

Spread the jam on toast, spoon it into Greek yogurt or on top of your breakfast porridge. If it is too tart for you, add honey or blended dates, which are high in natural sugars.

250g blueberries

250g of your favourite seasonal fruit – strawberries, raspberries, rhubarb, plums, etc.

seeds from ½ vanilla pod

1 tbs white chia seeds

Place the fruit and vanilla seeds in a small pan, add 2 tbs water and gently simmer for about 10 minutes until the fruit is soft and the liquid has evaporated. Add the chia seeds, mix and leave to cool. It will take on a jammy consistency and works brilliantly as a sugar-free, very healthy replacement for jam. Stored in the fridge in an airtight container, it will keep for up to a week.

Ground-seed sprinkle

takes 5 minutes

Every few days, I grind up seeds, such as those listed below, and then use them in almost all my cooking – sprinkled on porridge, added to smoothies, scattered over soups, salads or grilled fish, added as a thickener to soups and casseroles, added to home-made flapjacks, cookie sprinkles, on to a carrot cake . . . Seeds really are very versatile and nutritious, and can provide a boost of energy, so do make use of them wherever you can. Once ground, store the mix in the fridge to keep the seeds as fresh as possible.

1 tbs sesame seeds
1 tbs pumpkin seeds
1 tbs sunflower seeds
1 tbs hemp seeds

Place all the seeds in a Nutribullet or blender and blitz until they look like sand. The longer you blitz, the finer they become.

Nut butter

makes 1 small jar

takes 5 minutes + 30 minutes' soaking time for the nuts

This is a really useful way to add nut nutrition to soups and casseroles – or you can simply spread it on hot toast. If you feel you need a quick sweet treat, take a Medjool date, cut it in two and spread one half with a generous amount of nut butter and sandwich it back together. It's like a powerball but made in seconds and not so messy!

100g of your favourite raw nuts – peanuts, cashews, almonds, brazils, walnuts, hazelnuts, etc.

75–100ml warm water

pinch of salt

Place the nuts and warm water in a blender and leave to sit for 30 minutes, add the salt and then blend rapidly until smooth and creamy. The consistency will depend on your blender. A Nutribullet works best; a Magimix takes longer and even then may deliver a coarser blend. If you want a thinner nut butter, add a little more warm water to adjust. Always store in the fridge. It will keep for up to 5 days.

Nausea settlers

Although pregnancy is an exciting time, nausea and vomiting – also known as morning sickness – can be a really awful experience. No two cases are ever the same, but it is most common in the early stages of pregnancy when high levels of hormones are flooding your body.

Eating small quantities of food fairly frequently (the 'little and often' principle) can help, as can ginger, which acts to calm an irritated stomach by helping to neutralize stomach acid and relax the stomach muscles. Nibble on these easy-to-prepare recipes to ease your nausea and/or sickness.

Ginger and pineapple smoothie

serves 2

takes 15 minutes

5cm fresh ginger, peeled and chopped
¼ pineapple, peeled and cut into chunks
approx. 500ml coconut water

Place the chopped ginger, pineapple and coconut water in a Nutribullet or blender and blitz until completely smooth.

Carrot, turmeric and kale soup

serves 2

takes 40 minutes

Coconut oil is a good oil to cook with as it can be heated without releasing any dangerous chemicals and is therefore easier to digest. This nutrient-rich soup is wonderfully healing to the gut, so if you are suffering from heartburn or nausea this would be a really good choice.

1 tbs coconut oil
1 onion, diced
1 clove garlic, crushed
1 tsp ground turmeric, or 5cm grated if fresh
250g carrots, diced
1 litre vegetable or chicken stock
250g kale, chopped

Heat the coconut oil in a medium saucepan, add the onion and garlic and cook for 5 minutes or until soft. Add the turmeric and carrots, pour in the stock, bring to the boil then simmer for 30 minutes. Season and blend until smooth. Add the chopped kale, stir and simmer for 3 minutes before serving. If you prefer a totally smooth soup, add the kale before blending, cook for a further 5 minutes and then blend.

Oat and seed baked wafers

serves 2

takes 2.5 hours + 12 hours' soaking

These little wafers are delicious to nibble on their own or when served with dips, soups and cheese. Make a batch and enjoy them instead of shop-bought biscuits that may contain damaging fats, sugar and chemicals.

50g oats
50g sunflower seeds
50g pumpkin seeds
50g sesame seeds

1 tbs psyllium husks
sea salt and freshly ground pepper
2 tsp dried rosemary

Mix together the oats, sunflower, pumpkin and sesame seeds, cover with water and soak for 12 hours in a cool place. The next day, pre-heat the oven to 120°C, gas mark 1, drain the water through a fine sieve and return the ingredients to the bowl. Add the psyllium husks, seasoning, rosemary and 100ml of water and mix well. Leave to sit for 15 minutes, stirring from time to time. The psyllium will swell and absorb the water. Add a little more water if needed; the mixture should be able to hold its own shape.

Line a large baking sheet, approximately 36 × 36cm, with parchment, place the mixture on to the sheet and spread it out very thinly (the thinner the better) across the whole surface with a palette knife. Place in the oven and cook for 2 hours until dried and just golden. Allow to cool and then break into pieces. Store in an airtight container.

Yogurt and fruit lollies

serves 2

takes 20 minutes to prepare + 2 hours' freezing time

If your body's thermostat is out of kilter, these lollies could be just the answer to help you to cool off; not only that, they're good for you too. It's best to use seasonal fruit, but as a rule of thumb stronger-tasting fruits make tastier lollies. In the winter, try soaking dried fruits in a little hot water to soften them and then drain and blend. Dates work really well.

200g fruit, liquidized – strawberries, raspberries, blackberries,
**   blackcurrants, etc.**
100g Greek yogurt

Mix the liquidized fruit and yogurt together until evenly blended, then place into lolly moulds and freeze for at least 2 hours.

Barley, lemon and ginger water

makes 750ml

takes 20 minutes (+ 12 hours' soaking)

If you are feeling a bit under the weather, a cooling, calming glass of this tasty juice may help to settle an upset stomach. Barley is also known for its ability to flush out toxins and is one of the best natural remedies for urinary tract health.

100g barley
750ml water
10cm ginger, peeled and finely sliced
juice of 2 lemons
25g sugar

Rinse the barley well in cold water and drain. Then place the barley in a pan, cover with 750ml of water, add the sliced ginger and leave to sit in a cool place for 12 hours. Then bring to the boil and simmer for 15 minutes. Remove from the heat and leave to cool.

When cool, drain through a sieve, reserving the water. Add the lemon juice and sugar to the liquid, mix well and chill in a covered jug in the fridge. It will keep for a week.

Good foods to include in your diet

Whether pregnant or not, you should always aim to buy the best-quality food that your budget will allow. However, during your pregnancy it is even more important to remember that the food you eat can give you and your baby the best possible start to this new and exciting chapter in your life. See the chart opposite.

Shops and supermarkets have a wonderful array of healthy foods on offer, but try visiting your local farmers' market to find locally sourced foods if you can. (This can be fun, as there will usually be an artisan café or pop-up shop where you can enjoy a healthy breakfast or lunch while gathering some fresh-from-the-farm produce or other locally sourced foods.) If this is not an option for you, try to select outdoor-reared/free-range meats and line-caught fish whenever possible, and aim to cook seasonally if you can.

Remember, locally grown produce will be fresher and more nutritious than produce that has travelled hundreds, or even thousands, of miles. In fact, it's important to keep an eye on what looks fresh and appetizing. If an ingredient in your chosen recipe doesn't look good, the chances are it won't taste good either, so be prepared to adapt and improvise when cooking.

GOOD FOODS	
Lean red meat	Beef, lamb, venison
White meat	Chicken, turkey, game birds, pork
Fish	All fish, including oily fish such as salmon, mackerel and tuna (see note on pages 174–5 regarding tuna), and seafood, which should *always* be purchased from a reliable source. Seafood contains zinc, which is an important nutrient.
Vegetables	All vegetables are recommended (particularly dark-green vegetables), as they are an excellent source of fibre and vitamins.
Fruits	All fruits offer incredible health benefits and will give your diet an essential boost of fibre and vitamins.
Dairy	Greek yogurt, hard cheese, milk (in moderation)
Nuts, seeds, healthy oils	Nuts and seeds are a great source of protein, minerals, zinc and other essential nutrients. Try to include a range of healthy oils in your diet – olive, flax, hemp and coconut.
Grains, beans, pulses	These store-cupboard staples are inexpensive, nutritious and extremely versatile – perfect for those days when you can't face shopping.
Wholemeal and seeded breads	Adds essential fibre to the diet.

Foods to avoid

Apart from the foods already mentioned (such as liver, shark and swordfish, trans-fats, caffeine, alcohol, retinol supplementation, refined carbohydrates and artificial sweeteners), there are many other foods that should be avoided during pregnancy. These include foods that carry a risk of food-borne illness that could cause miscarriage, premature or stillbirth, or birth defects. There is a great deal of advice and literature on this subject, and the guidance is updated regularly (http://www.nhs.uk/Conditions/pregnancy-and-baby/Pages/foods-to-avoid-pregnant.aspx).

Salmonella is the most common cause of food poisoning and can be found in raw egg, uncooked poultry and shellfish. Eat hard-boiled eggs and check that chicken is cooked all the way through. If you have handled raw chicken, or indeed any raw meat, wash your hands and any utensils thoroughly. Only eat cooked shellfish.

Listeria is a bacteria that can be found in soft cheeses that have been mould-ripened, blue-veined cheeses, unpasteurized milk and milk products, and pâté. Packaged salads can also be a source of listeria, so wash the leaves thoroughly even if it says 'washed and ready to eat' on the packaging. Fruit and vegetables should also be washed well. Listeria can be destroyed by heat, so it is fine to eat the cheeses if they are thoroughly cooked. Ready meals should always be heated thoroughly and avoid those that do not require heating, such as ready-cooked quiches and meat pies.

Soft cheeses that can be eaten are cottage cheese, mozzarella, feta, cream cheese, paneer, ricotta, halloumi and goats' cheese.

Campylobacter can be contracted from poultry, unpasteurized milk and milk products (such as ice cream), soil and pets. Again, be careful to cook poultry thoroughly and do not contaminate kitchen areas, utensils and other food with the raw meat. If you have pets, always wash your hands after touching them and keep their food bowls separate to yours.

Toxoplasmosis can be contracted from cat faeces, so always wear gloves when gardening or cleaning out cat litter. Toxoplasmosis contracted during pregnancy can cause brain damage and blindness to unborn babies. Foods where it can be found are raw meat, cold cured meats such as salami, and unpasteurized milk and milk products. Cooking meats well, including cured meats, renders them safe.

Green or sprouting potatoes contain **alpha–solanine and alpha–chaconine**, which have been linked to neural-tube defects.

And Finally . . .

It has been my honour and my pleasure to accompany you through the most incredible, life-changing event in a woman's, and a man's, life. This has truly been a journey of discovery, from conception to birth and beyond, and I hope I have provided you with practical advice on exercise, nutrition and lifestyle that has enhanced your experience of pregnancy and enabled you to rapidly return to a healthy, normal life – although 'normal' will never be the same again!

Being active and eating well are key elements of the pregnancy journey, from pre-conception through to the post-partum period, and each new addition to any family brings a host of delights and challenges! Having made positive changes to your exercise, nutrition and lifestyle, you are now in a fabulous place to begin your new life as a mum. And remember, exercise and a healthy, balanced lifestyle are for life, not just for pregnancy!

I hope that you will take what you have learned from this book and continue to exercise safely and effectively, eat healthily and make positive lifestyle changes as you become a role model for your new baby.

I have thoroughly enjoyed writing this book and having the opportunity to join you, in some small way, on your journey of a lifetime.

I wish you every success in your future lives together as an active, healthy family.

August 2016

Acknowledgements

As with pregnancy, the production of this book, from conception to delivery and beyond, has only been possible with the support, commitment, dedication and hard work of an outstanding team of specialists. I would like to thank everyone who has been involved with *Bump It Up*, but I would particularly like to highlight the outstanding contribution of the following.

I would like to thank the team at Transworld Publishers, in particular my editor Brenda Kimber, who has been a shining light throughout the entire process, guiding me (and often pushing me!) in the right direction. Thanks also go to Ailsa Bathgate for her thorough and insightful review of the text; to Liane Payne for the fabulous illustrations; and design manager Phil Lord. Thanks also to Andy Allen for the wonderful jacket design, and to publicity manager Sarah Harwood for her critical work in promoting the book. It has been a true pleasure to work with such a professional, caring team.

I would like to thank two very special people: nutritionist Catherine Zabilowicz for her professional advice on nutrition and healthy eating, and food writer Fran Warde for her delicious recipes. I am indebted to them both for their guidance and support.

Special thanks to Andy Digweed and my management team at Sports Sphere. Andy and the team are a source of continual support and without their help this book would not have been possible.

As always, nothing that I achieve would be possible without my own very personal team – Penny, my wife, and my three children, Maya, Elise and Mitchell. Thank you.

Index

salmon cakes with chia seeds,
broccoli and cashew-nut stir-fry
202–3
broths
miso broth with vegetables and
udon noodles 194–5
super broths and Asian-style quick
soups 207–8
bruschetta topped with tinned
sardines, tomato and avocado
199
bulimia 4
bum lifts 66, 95
bump
during second trimester 80, 81, 111
during third trimester 107
and exercise 25, 26
butter bean, avocado and tomato
salad with feta 195–6
butternut squash: hot tuna butternut
Niçoise 204

C
cabbage
pearl barley and green
vegetable-style risotto with
added chicken shreds 197–8
rump steak ribbons with coconut
rice and vegetable stir-fry 200–1
cadmium 171
caesarean sections 140, 161–2
and exercise 26, 148, 152, 161–2,
165, 166
increasing your risk of 22, 173
post-partum 148, 152, 161–2, 165,
166
probiotics 184
reducing your risk of 26
caffeine 171

during pregnancy 182
effect on fertility 2, 3, 6, 10
and infertility 172
calcium 18, 180, 181
calf stretches 57
calories
during second trimester 36
post-partum 165
campylobacter 220
cannabinoids 12
carbohydrates 5, 6, 20, 36, 177,
182, 183
cardiovascular system
(baby's) 44
cardiovascular system (mother's)
changes to during pregnancy
18, 19
effects of exercise on 24, 25
carrot, turmeric and kale soup
214–15
cashew nuts: salmon cakes with chia
seeds, broccoli and cashew-nut
stir-fry 202–3
cat stretches 96
cat and extension 128
cell damage 5
centre of gravity 19, 39
post-partum 145, 155
second trimester 82, 88, 101, 107
third trimester 112, 113
cervix 138
cervical screening tests 14
cheese 220
butter bean, avocado and tomato
salad with feta 195–6
chemicals 175
chest
chest pain 27
chest stretch 55

chia seeds
  fresh fruit and chia-seed sugarless
    jam 211
  red berry, lemon and chia-seed
    smoothie 189
  salmon cakes with chia seeds,
    broccoli and cashew-nut stir-fry
    202–3
chicken 220
  ginger chicken soba noodles with
    bok choi and peas 201–2
  pearl barley and green
    vegetable-style risotto with
    added chicken shreds 197–8
cholesterol 18
clams 91, 96, 156
clothing
  and fertility 11
  sports clothing 49, 58
cocaine 13
coconut, banana and ginger
    smoothie 192
cod liver oil 177
cognitive behavioural therapy 8
colostrum 110
conception, increasing chances of 1, 2
  see also fertility; infertility
congestion 80, 110
connective tissue, effects of relaxin
    on 18, 63, 73, 93, 125, 160, 161
constipation 46, 79, 102, 110, 177
contact sports 48, 88
contractions, Braxton Hicks 111
cooling down 50, 115, 126
copper 181
core muscles
  core and split-ab workout 155–8
  effects of pregnancy on 17, 20
  first trimester 63–8

post-partum 152
second trimester 81
third trimester 112
core strength and stability exer-
    cises 24
  first trimester 64–8, 72
  post-partum 152–8, 164
  second trimester 92–7, 100, 103
  third trimester 124–33, 134
cortisol 8, 25, 172
cosmetics 175
couscous: Moroccan lamb with
    apricots, minted almond
    couscous and watermelon 205–6
cramps
  leg cramps 27, 80, 110, 146
  vaginal cramps 142
cravings 175–6
cross-training 59, 112, 113, 148
crying 81
cushion squeeze 67, 94, 157
cycling 58, 59, 112, 113, 148

D
dairy 188, 219
dance classes 113
dates: fruitjacks 210
deep-water walking 87
defecation, post-partum 143
dehydration 48, 49
depression
  during pregnancy 73
  and exercise 8, 16, 25
  postnatal depression (PND) 145,
    166–7
  post-partum 140
diabetes, gestational 22, 26, 40, 104,
    173, 182, 184–5
diaphragm 18, 20

first trimester 54–7
third trimester 115, 126–7, 136
foetus
core temperature 75
foetal development 44–5, 77–8, 103, 107–9
foetal macrosomia 40
foetal movements 27, 44–5, 78, 81, 108, 111
foetal programming 184
heart rate during exercise 74
folate 6, 75, 174, 179
folic acid 75, 174
follicle stimulating hormone (FSH) 7
food
food fetishes 47
foods to avoid 220–1
good foods to include in your diet 218–19
forgetfulness 81, 111
front arm lifts 123
fruit 6, 174, 177, 183, 219, 220
fresh fruit and chia-seed sugarless jam 211
sunrise fruit salad with spiced ground-seed sprinkle 193
yogurt and fruit lollies 216–17
fruitjacks 210

G
gait 108, 134–5
gender 137
ginger 183
barley, lemon and ginger water 217
coconut, banana and ginger smoothie 192
ginger and pineapple smoothie 214
ginger chicken soba noodles with bok choi and peas 201–2

gingivitis 80, 111
glucagon 25
glucose 25
glycogen 25
grains 219
greens 6
growth hormone 19, 25
gum sensitivity 80, 111

H
haemorrhoids 80, 102, 143
hair loss 140, 143, 168
hamstring stretch 56
hands (baby's) 44
headaches 22, 27, 46, 73, 80, 110, 125
heart (baby's)
development of 44
heart rate when mother exercising 74
heart (mother's)
changes to during pregnancy 18, 19
heart rate during exercise 24, 30–2, 50
heart rate during pregnancy 18, 36, 80
heartburn 21, 22, 46, 79, 110
heart rate monitors 32
heavy-metal toxicity 171–2
heel taps 52, 117
hormones
during first trimester 45
during second trimester 81
effect of cannabinoids on 12
effect of lifestyle on 7
effects of exercise on 25
levels during pregnancy 18, 19
post-partum 140, 143, 145, 162, 168–9
stress hormones 8
see also oestrogen; relaxin, etc.
human chorionic gonadotrophin (HCG) 18, 45, 140

lipids 18, 19
listeria 220
lochia 142, 148, 164, 165
lollies, yogurt and fruit 216–17
lunches 194–9
lunges 61, 122, 150
    lunge and bicep curl 85
    reverse lunge and bicep curl 62
    side lunges 56
lungs (baby's) 108, 137
luteinizing hormone 8, 19
lycopene 6

M
macronutrients 5, 174, 175–81
magnesium 181
mangoes: sunrise fruit salad with
    spiced ground-seed sprinkle 193
marching 51, 116
marijuana 12
meat 177, 219, 220, 221
medication and fertility 8, 13, 73, 175
melons: sunrise fruit salad with
    spiced ground-seed sprinkle 193
men
    age and fertility 11–12
    alcohol and fertility 7
    exercise and sperm count 4–5
    and healthy lifestyles 34–5
    improving fertility 6, 11
    smoking and fertility 7–8
    sperm count 4, 5, 12
    sperm motility 12, 14
    stress and fertility 8
    tight clothing and fertility 11, 12
menstruation 4, 9
mental health 73
    benefits of exercise on 16, 25
    depression 8, 16, 25, 73

postnatal depression (PND) 145,
    166–7
post-partum 140, 146, 163
metabolic system 35–6
    changes during pregnancy 19, 20
    during first trimester 48, 50
    effects of exercise on 25
methylfolate 174
Mexican refried beans with spinach
    and poached egg 196–7
microbiota 184–5
micronutrients 5, 174
    micronutrient deficiency
        171, 172
milk 220, 221
milk production, and exercise 165
mindfulness 8, 73, 136
mint: Moroccan lamb with apricots,
    minted almond couscous and
    watermelon 205–6
miscarriages 181, 182
miso broth with vegetables and udon
    noodles 194–5
mitochondria 75
mobile phones 14
moods 25
    low moods 73, 74
    mood swings 47, 81, 111, 143
    post-partum 144
morning sickness 100, 183
    nausea settlers 214–17
Moroccan lamb with apricots, minted
    almond couscous and water-
    melon 205–6
mother and baby classes 163
movements, foetal 44–5, 78, 81,
    108, 111
muesli, home-made nut and seed 191
multivitamins 6

push-ups 84
pyridoxine 178